I0840965

Introduction

I'll get right to it in this volume. If you have read the previous volumes in the series, then you and I both know it is high time that I "cut to the chase" and provide these lists of the very best natural sources of not only the 41 essential nutrients identified by the FDA for which they provide an RDA – Recommended Daily Allowance, but also for the variety of other nutrients found in natural foods that provide tremendous health benefits as well, not only as daily nutrition, but also as curative/preventatives that can help us keep from getting sick and also HEAL us after we do get sick.

I will cover the remedials (those foods or their byproducts, like all-natural extracts, juices, etc.) that have amazing beneficial properties like aloe vera, in upcoming volumes. This book will focus primarily on the 41 recognized essential nutrients and many others that should be included in a regular natural whole foods diet, if not daily, definitely at least once a week.

I am going to provide some websites a bit of free publicity because they offer a lot of excellent information and even though I have been studying the whole healthy diet issue for over 30 years, they have taught me plenty as I peruse through their web pages confirming each nutrient's health benefits and the terrible consequences of chronic deficiency.

The two main complaints that I always hear are: 1) It costs too much to eat healthy and 2) Health foods taste terrible. On the issue of taste, there is no question that a bacon and eggs breakfast is tastier to me than a bowl of old-fashioned oatmeal no matter how I try to dress it up and I do cheat on occasion and have a big greasy breakfast like that, but the whole key to everything is MODERATION.

I know it is one of the worst clichés ever, but you are what you eat. But there is a LOT more to it than that. Being healthy is a conscious choice that involves a lot of moving parts, not just the kinds of food a person eats, but also the AMOUNTS, and the SCHEDULE of meals and exercise is a critical part of the program that many people choose to ignore. Inactivity however, is a serious KILLER. Not only does it reduce the need for calories such that most people eat far more calories that they need, which causes the body to STORE all of those extra calories as body fat, but it also weakens the cardiovascular system making the person susceptible to a whole plethora of terrible diseases ranging from atherosclerosis to congestive heart disease and most of these lead to heart attack, stroke, and death. With cancer and heart disease conspiring to claim over 700,000 lives each year, most of which are PREVENTABLE, it is high time that we all start watching out for ourselves because it looks like no one else is going to do it!

I'll split this up into animal products, then plant foods. In the next chapter I provide the cross reference, so you can look up a specific nutrient and then see which superfoods will provide it. The list of the superfoods attempts to set everything to 1 oz. (28.35g.) Based on the amounts of carbohydrates and proteins this equates to anywhere from 0 calories for foods devoid of carbohydrates and proteins, to an upper limit of about 255 cal. per oz. of pure saturated animal fat.

DEFINITION OF A SUPERFOOD

The term "superfood" has indeed become a mainstay buzz word in the health and wellness field and we all get the general gist of the term, but I would like to be clear about what foods qualify as superfoods because I am going to list a lot of them and to many people they don't seem to be superfoods at all.

BASIC DEFINITION:

SUPERFOOD – Any food that in a "reasonable" amount will provide 100% of the RDA of at least one of the 41 identified essential nutrients OR is the best source of at least one identified nutrient that can make a significant contribution to your health.

In other words, "A nutrient that can make a significant contribution to your health," is one that does not currently have an RDA value established for it, but which can and will promote better health like lycopene or lutein, both close relatives to beta-carotene which is not actually Vitamin A, but is the only source of the vitamin for many people.

Two other factors of great significance are: 1) Portion size, and 2) Availability. I will mention some foods that are not very easy to find in your local grocery store and this makes them "low availability" foods. For example, some foods like Gac, a Vietnamese fruit, are nearly impossible to find. It certainly is a superfood, but that information is of no value if you can't ever find any to eat. On the other hand, tomatoes are almost year-round fixtures in every grocery store in the country and very likely worldwide. This makes them a superfood due to their high availability and high lycopene content.

When I look up "Foods high in X" and a given food like Eggs is listed as containing 10%DV (Daily Value – some websites define a value different from the RDA, usually higher, and so they use this term instead) then I consider the food and the information to be worthless. I am not going to eat eggs by the dozen, nor am I going to chart all 41 nutrients daily. For that I will just swallow a bowl full of natural extract supplements and be done with it.

But we are not stuck in a space capsule either, so we don't have to depend on a George Jetson diet of pills in order to get everything we need; there are whole natural foods, that despite the high intensity agricultural industry that keeps pumping them out of long dead dirt, still contain enough nutrients to keep us healthy without having to eat them by the bushel.

As such my definition of "superfood" is a bit more relaxed than most with respect to the nutritional content: one essential or highly beneficial nutrient and in a reasonable portion size and easily available in most stores at least part-time during the year, will get the food into this list. However, there are highly available foods with reasonable portion sizes that provide two or even more essential nutrients in at least 100% RDA quantities: shouldn't those be the true superfoods? I guess I would have to call them the "superduperfoods" and I will call your attention to these special nutrient packed foods; they are those foods that get into what I call my "Top Recommended Superfoods" list.

All foods include their ORAC Score as well. See Antioxidants in the next chapter for details.

ANIMAL PRODUCTS – SEAFOOD

Landlubbers in the middle states might not be used to having seafood but I assure you that fish and shellfish are loaded with essential nutrients often those that are extremely hard to find in sufficient quantities from any other source such as Zinc and Selenium. And while some nuts are loaded with alpha-Linoleic acid – one of the Omega-3 fatty acids – there are NO OTHER SOURCES of DHA and EPA Omega-3 fatty acids except for seafood and those are ESSENTIAL NUTRIENTS that you must get in your daily diet and they are NOT micronutrients either – you need a LOT of them (somewhere between 500mg and 1000mg) on a daily basis to maintain optimum and THRIVE-LEVEL health. These Omega-3's are critical for cardiovascular system health and brain function too. So break out the canned tuna fish and go for it!

*ATLANTIC MACKEREL** (Wild-caught) – (#1 SOURCE OF OMEGA-3 DHA and EPA) - This is the first of the fish, and if all you ever eat for the rest of your life is fish, you will be joining the Japanese who are, as a society, the healthiest on planet Earth. Mackerel makes this list for one reason: Omega-3 fatty acids DHA and EPA, but it has a lot more in it than that.[1]

ORAC Score: 120

1 OZ. CONTAINS:		%DV
Calories	57.4	3%
From Fat	35.1	(1)
From Protein	22.2(5.2g)	10%
Saturated Fat	0.9g	5%
Cholesterol	19.6mg	7%
Total Omega-3 fatty acids	748mg	(1)
Total Omega-6 fatty acids	61.3mg	(1)
Water	17.8g (63% by weight)	(1)
Vitamin D3	101 IU	25%

Niacin	2.5mg	13%
Vitamin B12	2.4mcg	41%
Selenium	12.3mcg	18%

Atlantic mackerel is a significant source of Complete Protein (2) and is the highest density source of the Omega-3 fatty acids DHA and EPA. A 5 oz. serving will provide: 50%DV of Complete Protein, 3,500mg of DHA/EPA Omega-3 fatty acids (all research to date suggests that you cannot "overdose" on the Omega-3's), 125%DV of Vitamin D3 (the good form that your own skin makes,) 65%DV Niacin, 205%DV Vitamin B12, and 90%DV Selenium.[2]

*TUNA (light, chunk, canned in water) – This superfood is readily available in any grocery store and is loaded with nutrients and the Omega-3 fatty acids as well as Complete Protein. Tuna fish is loaded with Niacin, Vitamin B12 and selenium (most fish provide both iodine and selenium which the thyroid must have and this is why I believe that all modern humans are descendents of a group of ancient humans that depended on fish for survival; we are all descendents of ancient fish-eating humans.)

ORAC Score: 90

1 OZ. CONTAINS:		%DV
Calories	32.5	2%
From Fat	2.1	(1)
From Protein	30.4(7.1g)	14%
Saturated Fat	0.1g	0%
Cholesterol	8.4mg	3%
Total Omega-3 fatty acids	78.7mg	(1)
Total Omega-6 fatty acids	2.5mg	(1)
Water	20.9g (74% by weight)	(1)
Niacin	3.7mg	19%
Vitamin B6	0.14mg	10%
Vitamin B12	0.8mcg	14%
Selenium	22.5mcg	32%

A 5 oz. serving will provide 70%DV of Complete Protein (2), 400mg of DHA/EPA Omega-3 fatty acids, 95%DV Niacin, 50%DV Vitamin B6, 70%DV Vitamin B12, 160%DV Selenium.[1][3][4][5]

*SALMON (Wild-caught) This is the TOP RECOMMENDED SUPERFOOD of the fish. Salmon is loaded with essential nutrients as well as the powerful antioxidant called astaxanthin (astuh-ZAN-thin) which is 6,000 TIMES more potent than Vitamin C; the redder the meat, the higher the astaxanthin content.[1][4][5][6][7][8]

ORAC Score: 30

1 OZ. CONTAINS:		%DV
Calories	42.8	2%
From Fat	18.3	(1)

From Protein	24.5(6.1g)	12%
Saturated Fat	0.3g	1%
Cholesterol	17.9mg	6%
Total Omega-3 fatty acids	316mg	(1)
Total Omega-6 fatty acids	22.4mg	(1)
Water	21g (74% by weight)	(1)
Niacin	2.3mg	11%
Pantothenic acid	0.47mg	9.3%
Biotin	1.5mg	(2)
Vitamin B12	2.2mcg	36%
Vitamin D3	150 IU	37%
Selenium	8.4mcg	12%

A 5 oz. serving of wild-caught salmon provides 60%DV Complete Protein(2), 1,580mg of DHA/EPA Omega-3 fatty acids, 55%DV Niacin, 47%DV Pantothenic acid, 7.5mg Biotin (1000%DV for adult men,) 180%DV Vitamin B12, 185%DV Vitamin D3, 60%DV Selenium plus it is one of the best sources of astaxanthin.

*SARDINES (canned in oil) – (#1 SOURCE OF VITAMIN B12) This is another fish in the TOP RECOMMENDED SUPERFOODS list. If all they provided was the Vitamin B12, that would be enough to make the list, but they are also an excellent source of several other essential nutrients as well.[1][4][5][9]

ORAC Score: est. 30

1 OZ. CONTAINS:		%DV
Calories	58.2	3%
From Fat	28.9	(1)
From Protein	29.4(6.9g)	14%
Saturated Fat	0.4g	2%
Cholesterol	39.8mg	13%
Total Omega-3 fatty acids	414mg	(1)
Total Omega-6 fatty acids	992mg*	(1)
Water	16.7g (59% by weight)	(1)
Vitamin B12	2.5mcg	42%
Vitamin D3	76.2 IU	19%
Calcium	107mg	11%
Phosphorus	137mg	14%
Selenium	14.8mcg	21%

* From the oil they are packed in

Sardines are a significant source of CHOLESTEROL (as are ALL fish, by the way.) If you are suffering from high cholesterol issues then read "Vol. 6 Controlling Cholesterol Without Drugs."

A five ounce serving of Sardines provides 70%DV Complete

Protein(2), 2070mg of Omega-3 DHA and EPA, 210%DV Vitamin B12, 95%DV Vitamin D, 55%DV Calcium (very difficult daily requirement to fulfill from whole natural foods) 70%DV Phosphorus (also hard to fulfill) 105% Selenium.

***OYSTERS** (wild eastern, canned, #1 SOURCE OF ZINC) – There really is only ONE superfood that can load you up on Zinc in a reasonable portion size: oysters. Many folks might think they are disgusting, but I am a Florida boy born and raised and if it comes from the sea it is definitely on the menu and oysters are no exception to that rule. This might be a bit of a weird food item for most people but most well stocked grocery stores do carry them and they are not particularly expensive canned and luckily it does not take much to meet your daily requirement. Once you open that can however, there is no turning back. If it spoils it can make you really sick so divvy up the contents of the can in ziplock bags and throw them in the freezer QUICKLY to stave off the growth of those harmful bacteria. No ORAC score available.

1 OZ. CONTAINS:		%DV
Calories	19.3	1%
From carbohydrate	4.6	(1)
From Fat	6.2	(1)
From Protein	8.4(2.0g)	4%
Saturated Fat	0.2g	1%
Cholesterol	15.4mg	5%
Total Omega-3 fatty acids	147mg	(1)
Total Omega-6 fatty acids	13.7mg	(1)
Water	23.8g (84% by weight)	(1)
Vitamin B12	5.4mcg	89%
Copper	1.2mg	62%
Selenium	10.0mcg	14%
Zinc	25.5mg	170%

JUST ONE oz of wild oysters contains 170%DV Zinc, 89%DV Vitamin B12, 62%DV Copper and 14%DV Selenium. Oysters have the highest concentration of Zinc of any practical and available food source.[10][11]

***CLAMS** – (canned in brine, BEST SOURCE OF IRON) - Most folks who don't live in the "Nor-east" only get clams from canned New England Clam Chowder. However, most of these products have so few of them in the can that it should really be called clam-flavored potato chowder. But that's alright because they do sell canned clams in the canned meats section of most well stocked grocery stores and those little fellows will do the trick. The best way I have found to serve them is to buy 1 can of condensed clam chowder, one can of ready-to-eat clam chowder and one can of clams and dump all three into a pot mix them up and bring them to a boil with the lid on and the stove burner on low heat to keep it from burning on the bottom. No ORAC score available.

1 OZ. CONTAINS:		%DV
Calories	41.4	2%
From Carbohydrate	6.0	(1)
From Fat	4.9	(1)
From Protein	30.5(7.2g)	14%
Saturated Fat	0.1g	<1%
Cholesterol	18.8mg	6%
Total Omega-3 fatty acids	111mg	(1)
Total Omega-6 fatty acids	9.0mg	(1)
Water	17.8g (63% by weight)	(1)
Vitamin B2 (Riboflavin)	0.1mg	7%
Vitamin B3 (Niacin)	0.9mg	5%
Vitamin B12	27.7mcg	461%
Copper	0.2mg	10%
Iron	7.8mg	43%
Manganese	0.2mg	14%
Phosphorus	94.6mg	9%
Potassium	176mg	5%
Selenium	13.6mcg	19%
Zinc	0.8mg	5%

A 6.5 serving (the contents of a typical can of chopped wild clams) contains 91%DV Complete protein(2), 45%DV Riboflavin, 32%DV Niacin, 3000%DV Vitamin B12 (not a typo – they are really loaded with B12) 65%DV Copper, 280%DV Iron, 91%DV Manganese, 58%DV Phosphorus, 32%DV Potassium, 123%DV Selenium, 32% Zinc and all for about 270 calories (without the rest of the soup involved of course.) You cannot find a more readily available source of natural Iron in a convenient, low calorie, low fat, and inexpensive food. I have a small bowl of clam chowder with my lunch salad every day of the week.[4][5][12][13]

ANIMAL PRODUCTS – LAND ANIMALS

*LAMB (avg. of various cuts, lean, domestic) – Lamb is definitely in the TOP RECOMMENDED SUPERFOODS list. It is loaded with essential nutrients and is the best land animal "true" meat as far as the variety and amounts of those nutrients in it. No ORAC score.

1 OZ. CONTAINS:		%DV
Calories	68.0	3%
From Fat	47.1	(1)
From Protein	20.9(4.9g)	10%
Saturated Fat	2.3g	11%

		%DV
Cholesterol	19.6mg	7%
Total Omega-3 fatty acids	92.4mg	(1)
Total Omega-6 fatty acids	305mg	(1)
Water	17.7g (63% by weight)	(1)
Riboflavin	1.3mg	76%
Vitamin B12	0.9mcg	15%
Selenium	5.5mcg	8%
Zinc	2.2mg	15%

Lamb is loaded with Vitamin B2 – Riboflavin and many people are suffering from chronic deficiency in this critical nutrient. Lamb is also a significant source of Zinc (chronic deficiency is also wide spread and a serious health issue.)[11][14][15]

A five oz. serving provides 50%DV Complete Protein (2) 380%DV Riboflavin, 75%DV Vitamin B12, 40%DV Selenium, 75%DV Zinc.

***BEEF LIVER** – (TOP LAND ANIMAL FOOD) Beef liver provides more vitamins and minerals than any other form of meat. For those of us who don't particularly like it, it can be a challenge to add it to our regular eating regimen. I will include a natural whole food diet recipe/cookbook in this series.

ORAC Score: 710

1 OZ. CONTAINS:		%DV
Calories	37.8	2%
From Carbohydrate	4.3	
From Fat	9.2	(1)
From Protein	24.3(5.7g)	11%
Saturated Fat	0.3g	2%
Cholesterol	77.0mg	26%
Total Omega-3 fatty acids	2mg	(1)
Total Omega-6 fatty acids	89mg	(1)
Water	19.8g (69% by weight)	(1)
Vitamin A (Retinol)	4732 IU	95%
Vitamin B2 (Riboflavin)	0.8mg	45%
Vitamin B3 (Niacin)	3.7mg	18%
Pantothenic acid	2.0mg	20%
Vitamin B6 (Pyridoxine)	0.3mg	15%
Vitamin B9 (Folate)	81.2mcg	20%
Vitamin B12	16.6mcg	277%
Choline	93.3mg	17%
Copper	2.7mg	137%
Iron	1.4mg	8%
Phosphorus	108mg	11%

Selenium	14.8mcg	21%

Beef liver is very high in CHOLESTEROL.

A FOUR oz. serving contains 44%DV Complete Protein (2), 104%DV CHOLESTEROL, 380%DV Vitamin A, 180%DV Riboflavin, 72%DV Niacin, 80%DV Pantothenic acid, 60%DV Vitamin B6, 80%DV Folate, 1108%DV Vitamin B12 (very dense source of B12) 68%DV Choline, 548%DV Copper (can be toxic in extremes) 32%DV Iron (people think they get enough Iron from beef liver; it would take nearly a POUND a day and that would bring far too much cholesterol and copper) 44%DV Phosphorus, 84%DV Selenium.[4][14][16][17][18][19]

TURKEY (ground) – Turkey makes the list because it is highly available year round in most grocery stores across the nation. It also brings Complete Protein and a few other essential nutrients as well. Turkey protein does contain Tryptophan, an essential amino acid, and contrary to popular belief it DOES NOT CAUSE drowsiness at all. Drastically overeating turkey at Thanksgiving can bring a lot of LACTIC ACID (highest concentration in the dark meat) which can lead to this effect, but NOT the TRYPTOPHAN. Incidentally chicken has a higher concentration of Tryptophan than turkey and the lore never accuses chicken of having this effect because it DOESN'T. Furthermore, EVERY CELL IN YOUR BODY is loaded with Tryptophan too, it is a basic construction material found in ALL animal proteins.

ORAC Score: Est. 600

1 OZ. CONTAINS:		%DV
Calories	41.7	
From Fat	20.9	(1)
From Protein	20.9(4.9g)	10%
Saturated Fat	0.6g	3%
Cholesterol	22.1mg	7%
Total Omega-3 fatty acids	30.8mg	(1)
Total Omega-6 fatty acids	504mg	(1)
Water	20.2g (71% by weight)	(1)
Vitamin B3 (Niacin)	1.0mg	5%
Vitamin B6	0.1mg	5%
Selenium	5.3mcg	8%

A FIVE oz. serving of Turkey contains 25%DV Niacin, 25%DV Vitamin B6 and 40%DV Selenium which is otherwise difficult to find in most foods other than fish and nuts.[5][20]

ANIMAL PRODUCTS - DAIRY

While these are all technically SECONDARY FOODS that were added to our diet recently (in our evolutionary timeline; about 15,000 to 35,000 years ago) and lactose intolerance is on the rise because of this, dairy products make the superfoods list for ONE very important reason: they are the ONLY natural whole food sources of calcium in sufficient quantities on a daily basis to satisfy our rather large need for this critical mineral. We all know that we need calcium for our bones and teeth, but did you know that it is also used in the construction and maintenance of arteries and veins or that it is involved in our brain chemistry?

And just because you have stopped growing, that doesn't mean that you no longer need calcium because these other bodily systems need constant and large supplies of it daily. When you come up short, the bones will pull it from their own structures and release it into the bloodstream for these other critical uses and THAT is exactly why osteoporosis and other related bone degenerative diseases have become EPIDEMIC. Be sure you get at least the 100% RDA of calcium from natural whole foods because most supplements are all basically powdered ROCKS (calcium carbonate – LIMESTONE, calcium sulfate – GYPSUM or PLASTER-OF-PARIS, and calcium phosphate – CONCRETE) and we do NOT digest rocks. Furthermore, these supplements do not provide you with Vitamin D3, Magnesium, Vitamin K and Lysine (one of the nine essential amino acids found in all Complete Proteins) ALL of which are also needed by the body in order to be able to properly handle that Calcium. Excesses of Calcium without these helpers can and will lead to serious problems like plaque build up in the arteries and veins (atherosclerosis) as well as kidney stones because the kidneys will see the need to remove all of that excess unused calcium floating around in the blood.

If you are lactose intolerant or avoiding dairy, then the best artificial sources of Calcium are in the form CALCIUM CITRATE. And if you take 1000mg daily (the 100% RDA amount) then you must also make sure that you are taking 100% RDA amounts of Magnesium, Vitamin K, Vitamin D3 and Lysine so that the body can properly absorb and USE that calcium. Personally, I would rather eat cheese and the natural whole food sources of all of those helpers and never have to worry about it.

***CHEESE, PARMESAN or ROMANO** (whole, chunk, BEST SOURCE OF CALCIUM) – While grated Parmesan (or Romano) cheese have the same nutrient content, it is difficult to measure out and consume at least three ounces of it which is what you need on a daily basis to satisfy your need for Calcium.
ORAC Score: est. 80

1 OZ. CONTAINS:		%DV
Calories	110	5%
From Carbohydrate	3.4	
From Fat	63.6	(1)
From Protein	42.7(10g)	20%
Saturated Fat	4.6g	23%
Cholesterol	19.0mg	6%

Total Omega-3 fatty acids	83.1mg	(1)
Total Omega-6 fatty acids	76.2mg	(1)
Water	8.2g (29% by weight)	(1)
Calcium	331mg	33%
Phosphorus	194mg	19%
Selenium	6.3mcg	9%
Zinc	0.8mg	5%

Solid Parmesan or Romano cheese are very similar in nutrient content and are a significant source of excellent natural forms of calcium. A THREE oz. serving contains 60%DV Complete Protein (2) 100%DV Calcium (#1 source of any available food) 57%DV Phosphorus (an excellent source of this and we need a lot of it too) 27%DV Selenium and 15%DV Zinc. Keep this small amount of Zinc in mind if you add solid Parmesan or Romano cheese to your daily eating regimen like I have. It allows you to pursue just 85%DV of Zinc in other foods instead of all 100%.[11][21][22]

***CHEESE, SWISS** (whole, chunk, great source of CALCIUM) – If you cannot find whole solid Parmesan or Romano cheese at your store (and grated is just as good, you could put it into your salad, for example,) Swiss will do the trick. It has the second highest concentration of Calcium among the commonly available cheeses. ORAC Score: est. 60

1 OZ. CONTAINS:		%DV
Calories	106	5%
From Carbohydrate	5.8	
From Fat	68.4	(1)
From Protein	32.2(7.5g)	15%
Saturated Fat	5.0g	25%
Cholesterol	25.8mg	9%
Total Omega-3 fatty acids	98.5mg	(1)
Total Omega-6 fatty acids	174mg	(1)
Water	10.4g (37% by weight)	(1)
Vitamin B12	0.9mcg	16%
Calcium	221mg	22%
Phosphorus	159mg	16%
Selenium	5.1mcg	7%
Zinc	1.2mg	8%

Swiss Cheese is available in most stores year round and is an excellent source of Calcium, but it does have a lot of saturated fat and cholesterol making Parmesan and Romano cheeses highly preferable.

A FIVE oz. serving contains 75%DV Complete Protein (2) 80%DV Vitamin B12 (an excellent source of most of the NATURAL FORM of this vitamin that you need daily) 110%DV Calcium, 80%DV Phosphorus (you also need a lot of phosphorus and most dairy products bring a lot of it as well) 35%DV Selenium, and 40%DV Zinc. Because Swiss has a lot of Zinc in it, I have added it to my daily eating regimen as well. Between the Parmesan and the Swiss, they cover anywhere from 15% to 55% of my daily requirements for this mineral. I eat enough Pumpkin seeds to make up the difference with ease.[11][21][23][24]

YOGURT (plain, whole milk) – "Whole milk" is a marketing term introduced after the FDA imposed the rule that all store bought milk had to be homogenized and pasteurized. While the milk people were forced to do this they decided to skim most of the cream out to sell in other more expensive products like butter and cheese to get their money back from having to spend it on these processes. Because most of the cream was gone, people thought the milk tasted very bland and so the dairy people started calling it "Whole milk" to try to get people to buy it and drink it and the name stuck. When I ask most people these days what they think the fat content of modern whole milk is, they guess anywhere from 20% to 50%. Half and Half is about 20% to 40% and modern "whole milk" is actually about 3% to 5%. Organic Yogurt (made from grass-fed cattle milk) is loaded with iodine but hard to find. Yogurt is a dieter's best friend and it is loaded with Calcium.[21][23][25] ORAC Score: est. 60

1 OZ. CONTAINS:		%DV
Calories	17.1	1%
From Carbohydrate	4.9	
From Fat	8.0	(1)
From Protein	4.1(1g)	.2%
Saturated Fat	0.6g	3%
Cholesterol	3.6mg	1%
Total Omega-3 fatty acids	7.6mg	(1)
Total Omega-6 fatty acids	18.2mg	(1)
Water	24.6g (87% by weight)	(1)
Calcium	34mg	3%
Phosphorus	26.6mg	3%

TWO EIGHT oz. cups of yogurt daily provide 32%DV Complete Protein (2) 50%DV Calcium and 46%DV Phosphorus. These values are significantly higher in organic yogurt if you can find it.

HONORABLE MENTION – MILK (Whole or Skim) – While not an actual superfood, milk does have a lot of Calcium, an 8 oz serving brings about 30%DV and about the same percentage of Vitamin D3 as well. For most people milk may be their most available and cost effective way to get natural form Calcium. 8 oz Whole milk is about 150 calories and 2% Skim is about 120 calories. The difference is insignificant because whole milk is only about 3.5% fat anyway and the further processing REMOVES many fat soluble nutrients.

ANIMAL PRODUCTS – UNCATEGORIZED

There is nowhere else to put Cod Liver Oil, but it is definitely a "superfood" even though it is not technically a "food" at all. Nevertheless, it is a natural extract and it is certainly one of the healthiest "supplements" on Earth and even though it tastes horrible, I highly recommend it because it solves several important essential nutrient requirements quickly (if not easily!)

*COD LIVER OIL (crude, filtered) – Try to avoid highly processed products; the closer it is to what they squeeze out of the fish livers, the better. CLO is a tremendous source of the Omega-3's DHA and EPA as well as true animal form Vitamin A and Vitamin D3 which is the one we produce in our skin and all of these are NATURAL forms and not MANUFACTURED, ARTIFICIAL, FAKE forms. No ORAC Score.

1 TBSP (1/2 oz.) CONT:		%DV
Calories	122	6%
From Carbohydrate	0	
From Fat	122	(1)
From Protein	0(0g)	0%
Saturated Fat	3.1g	15%
Unsaturated fats	9.3g	(1)
Cholesterol	77mg	26%
Total Omega-3 fatty acids	2664mg	(1)
Total Omega-6 fatty acids	126mg	(1)
Water	0g (0% by weight)	(1)
Vitamin A (Retinol)	13500 IU	270%
Vitamin D3	1350 IU	338%

Just ONE TABLESPOON of COD LIVER OIL contains a huge amount of Omega-3 DHA and EPA, Vitamin A (one teaspoon should actually be enough) and a massive dose of natural form Vitamin D3 as well.[1][16][26][27]

HONORABLE MENTION – EGGS (EXCELLENT SOURCE OF CHOLINE AND THE B VITAMINS) – While high in fat and cholesterol, eggs are the most available source of choline.

PLANT SUPERFOODS – SEEDS AND NUTS

These foods are highly nutritious and some of the ONLY significant sources of Vitamin E which plays a pivotal role in PROTECTING the DNA in our cells and preventing it from being damaged. Damaged DNA is the very definition of CANCER and chronic deficiency in Vitamin E can very likely to lead to cancer. Most Americans DO NOT consume seeds and nuts of any kind on a regular basis except for peanuts in the form of peanut butter which does have some Vitamin E in it, but not enough to meet our 100% RDA DAILY REQUIREMENT. I believe that this is the #1 cause of many forms of cancer in the U.S. today.

There is no doubt that the seeds and nuts bring a lot of calories mainly because they are almost completely devoid of water and are instead solid chunks of protein and polyunsaturated fat which is where all of those calories are coming from but you must still try to incorporate them into you diet.

Do yourself a favor and ADD some seeds and nuts to your daily eating regimen to cover your 100% RDA of crucial Vitamin E and you will have taken a MAJOR STEP towards preventing the dreadful affliction called cancer. And, by the way, seeds and nuts are also the richest sources of many different minerals depending on the specific seeds and nuts that are otherwise very hard to get in 100% RDA amounts from any other kinds of foods.

***WALNUTS** (Top seed/nut source of Omega-3 fatty acid ALA) – There are plenty of varieties, but all of them have one thing in common: they are LOADED with alpha-Linoleic acid or ALA which is the ONLY Omega-3 fatty acid found in plants. We can convert some ALA into DHA and EPA (the animal Omega-3's) for ourselves IF we get some ALA in our diet. For those who do not eat fish very often, walnuts are the ONLY SIGNIFICANT HIGHLY AVAILABLE NATURAL WHOLE FOOD SOURCE of the Omega-3 fatty acids. How important are they? The FDA is currently studying them to determine the RDA for this ESSENTIAL NUTRIENT. ORAC Score: 13,541 (Excellent)

1 OZ. CONTAINS:		%DV
Calories	183	9%
From Carbohydrate	15.5	
From Fat	153	(1)
From Protein	14.8(4.3g)	9%
Saturated Fat	1.7g	9%
Cholesterol	0mg	0%
Phytosterols	20.2mg	(3)
Total Omega-3 fatty acids	2542mg	(1)
Total Omega-6 fatty acids	10666mg	(1)
Fiber	1.9g	8%
Water	1.1g (3% by weight)	(1)
Copper	0.4mg	22%
Manganese	1.0mg	48%

While Walnuts do bring a lot of Omega-3, they also bring a LOT of the Omega-6 fatty acids as well and it is believed that the higher the RATIO of Omega-3 to Omega-6, the better (too much Omega-6's appear to NEGATE the positive effects of the Omega-3's.) Therefore, you MUST incorporate FISH (which are relatively low

on the Omega-6's unless they are packed in vegetable oil) to your daily eating regimen. Walnuts are also a significant source of Manganese which is a vital mineral involved in many enzymes throughout the body. Watch your Manganese and Copper levels and try not to exceed them by far. Copper is critical but it can cause trouble in chronic excesses. Just 1 to 2oz. of Walnuts a day is sufficient to shore up both minerals and the Omega-3's in conjunction with a fish entrée as often as possible.[1][28][29]
***ALMONDS** (dry roasted, no salt, #1 SOURCE OF VITAMIN E) – Almonds are a superfood just for the Vitamin E, but they do bring a few KEY minerals that are otherwise hard to get in 100% RDA amounts as well.[30][31][32]
ORAC Score: 4454 (Very Good)

1 OZ. CONTAINS:		%DV
Calories	167	8%
From Carbohydrate	21.9	(1)
From Fat	124	(1)
From Protein	21.5(6.2g)	12%
Saturated Fat	1.1g	6%
Cholesterol	0mg	0%
Phytosterols	33.0mg	(3)
Total Omega-3 fatty acids	0mg	(1)
Total Omega-6 fatty acids	3542mg	(1)
Fiber	3.3g	13%
Water	0.7g (2% by weight)	(1)
Vitamin B2 (Riboflavin)	0.2mg	14%
Vitamin E	7.3mg	36%
Copper	0.3mg	16%
Magnesium	80.1mg	20%
Manganese	0.7mg	37%
Phosphorus	137mg	14%

A THREE oz. serving of almonds provides 39%DV Fiber, 108%DV Vitamin E (alpha-Tocopherol) 42%DV Riboflavin, 48%DV Copper, 60%DV Magnesium (very difficult to get in 100% RDA daily and very important) 111%DV Manganese, 42%DV Phosphorus.
***SUNFLOWER SEED KERNELS** – These are one of the TOP RECOMMENDED SUPERFOODS because they bring a LOT of essential nutrients. You can't go wrong adding them to your daily eating regimen. No ORAC score available.

1 OZ. CONTAINS:		%DV
Calories	163	8%
From Carbohydrate	27.5	(1)
From Fat	117	(1)

From Protein	18.8(5.4g)	11%
Saturated Fat	1.5g	7%
Cholesterol	0mg	0%
Phytosterols	0mg	(3)
Total Omega-3 fatty acids	19.3mg	(1)
Total Omega-6 fatty acids	9180mg	(1)
Fiber	2.5g	10%
Water	0.3g (1% by weight)	(1)
Vitamin B1 (Thiamine)	0.44mg	35%
Vitamin B2 (Riboflavin)	0.2mg	14%
Vitamin B3 (Niacin)	2.0mg	10%
Pantothenic acid	2.0mg	20%
Vitamin B6 (Pyridoxine)	0.2mg	11%
Vitamin B9 (Folate)	66.4mcg	17%
Vitamin E	7.3mg	36%
Copper	0.5mg	26%
Magnesium	36.1mg	9%
Manganese	0.6mg	30%
Potassium	238mg	7%
Phosphorus	323mg	32%
Selenium	22.2mcg	32%
Zinc	1.5mg	10%

Sunflower seeds are relatively devoid of trace phytonutrients (including the phytosterols) which is exactly why they taste rather bland, but they make up for that in the quantity of essential nutrients that they bring to the table. Due to high concentrations of copper and manganese, do not exceed an avg. or four to five oz. daily. A FIVE oz. serving contains: 175%DV Thiamine, 70%DV Riboflavin, 50%DV Niacin, 100%DV Pantothenic acid (Vitamin B5) 55%DV Vitamin B6, 85%DV Folate, 180%DV Vitamin E, 130%DV Copper (be careful with this one, don't consume excesses daily) 45%DV Magnesium (we do need as much magnesium as we can get) 150%DV Manganese (keep this as close to 100% avg. daily as possible as well) 35% Potassium (a critical nutrient that we need in HUGE quantities daily, sunflower seed kernels are denser in potassium than bananas) 160%DV Phosphorus (difficult to find in large quantities in any food, this and vitamin E make sunflower seeds a superfood) 160% Selenium (outstanding plant source of selenium which is rare outside of fish) 50%DV Zinc (another trace mineral hard to find in most foods.) [5][11][14][18][23][28][31][33][34][35][36][37][38][39][40]

PUMPKIN SEEDS (whole, roasted, #1 SOURCE OF ZINC) – We may not need a lot of Zinc compared to many other essential nutrients, but very few foods contain it in sufficient quantities to satisfy our DAILY 100% REQUIREMENT for it; Pumpkin seeds will cover it easily and for that reason alone, they are a superfood. No ORAC score available.

1 OZ. CONTAINS:		%DV
Calories	125	6%
From Carbohydrate	61.4	(1)
From Fat	45.5	(1)
From Protein	18.0(4.0g)	8%
Saturated Fat	1.0g	5%
Cholesterol	0g	0%
Phytosterols	0g	0%
Total Omega-3 fatty acids	21.6	(1)
Total Omega-6 fatty acids	2452	(1)
Fiber	0g	0%
Water	1.3g(4% by weight)	(1)
Copper	0.2	10%
Magnesium	73.4mg	18%
Manganese	0.1mg	7%
Potassium	257mg	7%
Zinc	2.9mg	19%

Pumpkin seeds are lower in calories than most of the other seeds and nuts and much lower in the Omega-6's too.[109]

A FIVE oz. serving brings 90%DV Magnesium (one of the best sources of this critical nutrient and we need a lot of it on a daily basis) 95% Zinc (good of this critical essential nutrient) 50%DV Copper and 35%DV Manganese. I include the Copper and Manganese values so you can make sure that you do not exceed their values by too much on an average daily basis. [11] [38] [41]

BRAZIL NUTS (whole kernel, #1 SOURCE OF SELENIUM) – For those who do not eat fish often and do not want to load up on the seeds and nuts (avoiding both food groups is a real problem, by the way) Brazil nuts can still solve your daily requirement of selenium easily.

ORAC Score: 1419

1 OZ. CONTAINS:		%DV
Calories	183	9%
From Carbohydrate	14.0	(1)
From Fat	155.8	(1)
From Protein	14(g)	%
Saturated Fat	4.2g	22%
Cholesterol	0mg	0%

Phytosterols	0mg	(3)
Total Omega-3 fatty acids	23.9mg	(1)
Total Omega-6 fatty acids	27350.0mg	(1)
Fiber	2.1g	8%
Water	4.6g (16% by weight)	(1)
Vitamin B1 (Thiamine)	0.2mg	10%
Vitamin E	1.6mg	8%
Copper	0.5mg	24%
Magnesium	105mg	26%
Manganese	0.3mg	17%
Phosphorus	203mg	20%
Potassium	184mg	5%
Selenium	536mcg	767%
Zinc	1.1mg	8%

Just TWO individual Brazil nut kernels will satisfy your daily requirement for Selenium; think of them as chewable all natural Selenium supplements.[5][42]

PISTACHIOS (whole, roasted) – These nuts make the list because they are an excellent source of Vitamin B6 (Pyridoxine) especially if you have not had any turkey for the day which is another excellent source of the vitamin.

ORAC Score: 7675 (Very Good)

1 OZ. CONTAINS:		%DV
Calories	160	6%
From Carbohydrate	31.4	(1)
From Fat	108	(1)
From Protein	20.7(6g)	12%
Saturated Fat	1.6g	8%
Cholesterol	0mg	0%
Phytosterols	59.9mg	(3)
Total Omega-3 fatty acids	73.4mg	(1)
Total Omega-6 fatty acids	3818mg	(1)
Fiber	2.9g	12%
Water	0.6g (2% by weight)	(1)
Vitamin B1 (Thiamine)	0.2mg	16%
Vitamin B6 (Pyridoxine)	0.4mg	18%
Copper	0.4mg	19%
Magnesium	33.6mg	8%
Manganese	0.4mg	18%
Phosphorus	136mg	14%
Potassium	292mg	8%

Getting an adequate supply of Vitamin B6 is challenging especially for those trying to avoid excessive calories. The two best sources by far are turkey and pistachios. Try to coordinate them into your daily diet so that you get as close to 100% RDA of this vitamin daily as you can. A FIVE oz. serving of pistachios contains 80%DV Thiamine, 90%DV Vitamin B6, 95%DV Copper, 40%DV Magnesium, 90%DV Manganese, 70%DV Phosphorus, 40%DV Potassium. Because these, like all nuts, are high in Copper and Manganese you should be careful when consuming several different kinds of nuts so you will NOT drastically exceed their RDA's. [18][23][28][33][36][38][39][43]

PLANT FOODS – LEAFY GREENS

I cannot possibly stress to you how IMPORTANT this FOOD GROUP is. Suffice it to say that raw edible leafy greens should be a MAJOR bulk component of your daily diet. They bring a little fiber (excellent for your digestion) and a lot of CHLOROPHYLL which is a proven liver DETOXIFIER. Even if you have never consumed alcohol in your life, that doesn't mean that your liver doesn't need ALL THE HELP IT CAN GET. And for the chlorophyll alone ALL leafy greens get honorable inclusion into the superfoods list; no questions asked. But that is only the beginning, many of these outstanding foods are loaded with additional nutrients like Vitamin K. Contrary to popular opinion, excesses of Vitamin K will NOT cause internal blood clotting leading to heart attacks or strokes. Deficiencies of Vitamin E which plays a key role in PREVENTING internal blood clots WILL cause them and result in heart attacks or strokes. Chronic deficiency of Vitamin K is nasty business and can lead to improper handling of calcium in the body including allowing it to form plaque on arterial walls called atherosclerosis which can and will lead to INTERNAL BLOOD CLOTS resulting in heart attack or stroke and even result in kidney stones. While I usually do not recommend exceeding the 100% RDA by extreme amounts, two to three times the RDA from all natural whole food sources like the leafy greens will not pose any health threat; on the contrary, nothing could be better for your liver and overall cardiovascular health.

*SPINACH (raw, BEST SOURCE OF VITAMIN K) – Popeye had it right, "If you wants to be strong, then eats your spinach." I can't complain about his grammar, mine is just about as bad but, you do need that Vitamin K and while most of the other dark leafy greens have plenty, Spinach is by far the best source and it happens to be loaded with chlorophyll which promotes liver health too. Best of all, it can be found year round in most grocery stores across the land. Add just one ounce to your lunch salad and you have gone a long way towards changing your diet to a far better one that will lead to a longer, healthier and happier life. If you like it boiled as a side dish for dinner then by all means do that too!
ORAC Score: 1687

1 OZ. CONTAINS:		%DV
Calories	6.4	<1%
From Carbohydrate	3.6	(1)
From Fat	0.9	(1)
From Protein	2.0(0.8g)	2%
Saturated Fat	0g	0%
Cholesterol	0mg	0%
Phytosterols	2.5mg	(3)
Total Omega-3 fatty acids	38.6mg	(1)
Total Omega-6 fatty acids	7.3mg	(1)
Fiber	0.6g	2%
Water	25.6g (90% by weight)	(1)
Vitamin A (beta-carotene)	2625 IU	53%
Vitamin C	7.9mg	13%
Vitamin B9 (Folate)	54.3mcg	14%
Vitamin K	135mcg	169%
Manganese	0.3mg	13%

Just ONE oz. contains 53%DV Vitamin A (as beta-carotene, a safe form) and 169%DV Vitamin K. Folate is difficult to acquire in 100% RDA amounts on a daily basis and you should try to avoid overdoing it with Manganese. [28][37][44][45][46]

***KALE** (raw, #1 SOURCE OF ZEAXANTHIN AND LUTEIN, #1 SOURCE of VITAMIN K) – If you have read "Vol. 4 Antioxidants, Fiber and More" then you already know that Zeaxanthin and Lutein are critical antioxidant relatives of beta-carotene found in the human eye and are suspected of being able to prevent eye health issues like cataracts as well as Macular Degeneration. But they do not appear to be effective in purified supplement forms. Kale is all-natural whole food and it is by far the richest source of both of these Xanthophylls. For those who don't like the taste, chop it up into a salad with chopped iceberg lettuce and hide it with a host of tasty additives like spiced up Oil and Vinegar dressing.
ORAC Score: 1770

1 OZ. CONTAINS:		%DV
Calories	14.0	1%
From Carbohydrate	10.1	(1)
From Fat	1.6	(1)
From Protein	2.3(0.9g)	2%
Saturated Fat	0g	0%
Cholesterol	0mg	0%
Phytosterols	2.5mg	(3)
Total Omega-3 fatty acids	38.6mg	(1)

Total Omega-6 fatty acids	7.3mg	(1)
Fiber	0.6g	2%
Water	23.6g (83% by weight)	(1)
Vitamin A (beta-carotene)	4305 IU	86%
Vitamin C	33.6mg	56%
Vitamin K	229mcg	286%
Manganese	0.2mg	11%

You might have noticed that Kale has even more Vitamin K than Spinach. The only reason I call spinach the best source of Vitamin K is because of its availability year round in all grocery stores either fresh or canned. A tossed salad with about 1 oz. of spinach and 1 oz. of Kale is ideal. You will get ALL of the Vitamin A for the day (as beta-carotene) and a megablast of Vitamin K which will NOT CAUSE INTENAL BLOOD CLOTTING – A LACK of Vitamin E and Vitamin K WILL CAUSE INTERNAL BLOOD CLOTTING. You also get a megablast of Chlorophyll from both of these leafy greens and Zeaxanthin and Lutein from the Kale. The Chlorophyll is a detoxifier for your liver and the Zeaxanthin and Lutein are connected to proper eye health.[16][44][46][47][48][49]

LETTUCE (GREAT "NET NEGATIVE CALORIE" FOOD) – This gives me an opportunity to expound upon this subject introduced in "Vol. 1 – Dieting and Losing Weight." Scientists are currently saying that there is no such food other than water; that all foods that bring even very few calories will not result in "burning more calories to digest them than they provide." I would like to take this opportunity to DISAGREE. You expend energy: 1) Chewing the food, 2) Manufacturing and losing saliva, 3) Manufacturing stomach fluid, 4) Reabsorbing the stomach fluid in the duodenum, 5) Absorbing those few calories in the intestines, 6) Peristalsis of the intestines (muscular contractions that move the food through the intestines,) 7) Heart beats to move the blood containing the absorbed nutrients from the capillaries of the intestines to the liver, 8) The work of the liver to reabsorb those nutrients and metabolize them and then release them back into the bloodstream at a later time, 9) Heart beats to move those nutrients out to the rest of the body. When all is said and done, the couple of calories you get from lettuce cannot possibly compensate for all of this WORK that has to be done handling the meal. Obviously, there are other things in most meals besides just lettuce, like tomatoes and shredded cheese and dressing (if we are talking about a salad) and those bring ample calories so the whole meal does result a net positive caloric intake. But straight lettuce plus a few onions and skinned cucumbers (all low calorie content foods) with nothing but a dash of IODIZED salt, a little red wine vinegar (NO OIL) and some fresh finely chopped spices WILL yield so few calories that if you stick to this formula plus a grapefruit (no sugar added) for breakfast, lunch and dinner, you will end up burning more calories during the day just to maintain your body temperature than you will get from this diet: NET NEGATIVE CALORIES for the day. And you WILL SHRINK, because your body will have no choice but to break into the fat reserves in order to have the calories to burn, just for normal simple operations. Before you try this however, I URGE you to read Vol. 1 – Dieting and Losing Weight." Net Negative Calorie diets CAN BE DANGEROUS and I cover far better options in that book.

ORAC Score: 2426 (Good)

1 OZ. CONTAINS:		%DV
Calories	3.9	<1%
From Carbohydrate	3.0	
From Fat	0.3	(1)
From Protein	0.6(0.3g)	1%
Saturated Fat	0g	14%
Cholesterol	0mg	0%
Phytosterols	2.8mg	(3)
Total Omega-3 fatty acids	14.6mg	(1)
Total Omega-6 fatty acids	5.9mg	(1)
Fiber	0.3g	1%
Water	26.8g (95% by weight)	(1)
Vitamin A (beta-carotene)	141 IU	3%
Vitamin K	6.7mcg	8%

A FIVE oz. serving (a rather large bowl) contains just 24.5 calories, 15%DV Vitamin A, and 40%DV Vitamin K. It will provide less than 10%DV of several other vitamins and a few minerals, but its main value is to take up space so you don't overdo it on the spinach and kale which should be added to this salad.[44][50][51]

CABBAGE – (EXCELLENT LOW CAL SIDE DISH, EXCELLENT SOURCE OF SULFUR, EXCELLENT SOURCE OF FOLATE) – This is another leafy green vegetable that is not technically a superfood in that it will not satisfy your RDA for any essential nutrients, but it will get you a LOT of sulfur; it is loaded with the glucosinolates (sulfur containing compounds) and while none of these are currently considered ESSENTIAL nutrients per se, that is only because the FDA feels that anyone eating a healthy diversified natural whole food diet will be getting enough sulfur compounds to satisfy their requirements of this vital mineral. But for those who have been on the packaged and processed foods DEATH diet for years, coming back to Earth's natural bounty can be confusing until you get your bearings. Cabbage is a source of chlorophylls, xanthophylls and a whole host of sulfur containing compounds and is also a relatively low calorie, alternative to the typical HEAVY, STARCHY, LOW-NUTRITIONAL-VALUE side dishes like potatoes (terrible) or rice (worse) or beans (worst.)

ORAC Score: 856 (boiled)

1 OZ. CONTAINS:		%DV
Calories	6.7	0%
From Carbohydrate	5.5	(1)
From Fat	0.4	(1)
From Protein	0.8(0.3g)	1%
Saturated Fat	0g	0%
Cholesterol	0mg	0%
Phytosterols	3.1mg	(3)
Total Omega-3 fatty acids	12.9mg	(1)
Total Omega-6 fatty acids	9.8mg	(1)
Fiber	0.6g	2%
Water	25.9g (91% by weight)	(1)
Vitamin C	14.3mg	24%
Folate	16mcg	4%
Potassium	68.9mg	2%

Just 4 oz. of Cabbage provides 100%DV Vitamin C (which most people don't know!) and 16%DV Folate (which are hard to come by in any food) and 8% Potassium (which is difficult to get enough of daily so every little bit helps.)[49][51][52]

Boiled up and slathered in real butter and plenty of black pepper is real deep south home cookin' like my dear old auntie used to make and really good for you too (I have cut back on the real butter, but a little won't kill you IF you are getting plenty of fiber and dark leafy greens to compensate.) Cole slaw is OFF the MENU because of the mayonnaise and trust me I LOVE mayo. But it is made with RAW EGGS which are TERRIBLE – they contain AVIDIN which binds primarily to Vitamin B7 – Biotin, but it also binds to the other B vitamins as well and prevents their absorption in the digestive tract. Eating Mayo and its kin (creamy salad dressings and dips) is like swallowing an ANTI-VITAMIN B NUKE – YOU LOSE ALL of the B vitamins in the meal before it, during it and after it. Avoid RAW EGGS and their products as if they contain radioactive rattlesnakes and you will be on the right track.

MUSTARD GREENS, COLLARD GREENS, TURNIP GREENS, ROMAINE LETTUCE, NAPA CABBAGE, ETC. (GREAT SOURCES OF CHLOROPHYLLS, VITAMIN K, and the XANTHOPHYLLS) – All of these dark leafy greens get their honorable mention here. While I won't give them their complete nutrient fact tables, suffice it to say that they are all definitely on the menu as superfoods containing a lot of chlorophyll which is an excellent liver detoxifier, Vitamin K that helps the body coordinate calcium: no vitamin K results in calcium build up on blood vessel walls (atherosclerosis) that can lead to heart attack and stroke as well as kidney stones (from excess free calcium in the blood being removed by the kidneys) as well as bone degenerative diseases like osteoporosis. So that huge CONCRETE tablet (calcium phosphate – it isn't exactly concrete, but it is not easily absorbed by the digestive system either) that many people are taking to try to prevent osteoporosis will give them heart attacks, strokes and kidney stones if they don't get plenty of NATURAL VITAMIN K along with it (artificial forms have been PROVEN to be TOXIC and should never be taken.) Those xanthophylls (yellow colored molecules that also perform photosynthesis) like Zeaxanthin and Lutein are powerful antioxidants AND natural forms are suspected of helping to prevent cataracts and macular degeneration eye disease. Finally, they are all extremely low calorie and zero cholesterol foods and even cooked they are still loaded up with all of these nutrients and should be the top choices for side dishes with any meal. So load up on those leafy greens! [44][46]

PLANT SUPERFOODS – EDIBLE RAW VEGETABLES
Obviously the leafy greens are edible raw, but there are many others including carrots, green beans, onions, scallions, celery, bell peppers, hot peppers, broccoli, cauliflower, etc. All of these plant foods that can be eaten raw are the PRIMARY FOODS that human beings evolved eating for hundreds of thousands to millions of years and our digestive systems are optimized to digest THESE FOODS and all others are technically lower in significance with the exception of animal meats which we were also eating along the way during our deep dark evolutionary past. Any plant food that must be cooked in order to MAKE it edible is a SECONDARY FOOD by definition; a food that was added after we tamed fire and accidentally discovered that cooking them transformed them from inedible stuff into edible foods. And our digestive systems are STILL ADJUSTING to this technological revolution that occurred about 15,000 to 35,000 years ago. Don't think so? Then why is lactose intolerance and gluten intolerance on the rise? Because in modern times, when random genes combine to create a new child, that person sometimes gets our basic digestive system which was not designed (did not evolve) to eat these normally inedible or unobtainable foods. These days however, our societies are far more forgiving than they were 15,000 years ago; if you couldn't stomach what was on the menu for the day, you went without and eventually you starved to death. Nowadays these folks simply go to the local grocery store and buy ALMOND MILK (NEVER SOY – THAT CRAP IS BAD FOR YOU) and gluten-free foods. There are only a few kinds of beans that you should eat and even then, only on rare occasion. If you never eat another bean and ELIMINATE SOY and its endless by-products found in practically every packaged and processed food in the U.S., you will have taken a MAJOR step toward living a longer, healthier and happier life.
*CARROTS** (BEST SOURCE OF VITAMIN A) – They don't have

the highest concentration of beta-carotene, but they are found in every grocery store in the land year round and just ONE medium sized carrot contains about 200% RDA of Vitamin A in the form of beta-carotene which is a FAR SAFER form to consume than pure Retinol or animal form Vitamin A. You can't go wrong eating carrots raw or cooked. The cooking does reduce the amount of beta-carotene in them by 30% or more, but the equivalent of two medium carrots sliced and cooked is still more than sufficient to fulfill your daily requirement of Vitamin A as beta-carotene in a SAFE ANTIOXIDANT form. Carrots are a highly nutritious low calorie and zero cholesterol snack too.

ORAC Score: 697 (raw) and 326 (boiled)

1 OZ. CONTAINS:		%DV
Calories	11.5	1%
From Carbohydrate	10.2	(1)
From Fat	0.6	(1)
From Protein	0.7(0.3g)	1%
Saturated Fat	0g	0%
Cholesterol	0mg	0%
Phytosterols	0mg	(3)
Total Omega-3 fatty acids	0.6mg	(1)
Total Omega-6 fatty acids	32.2mg	(1)
Fiber	0.8g	3%
Water	24.7g (87% by weight)	(1)
Vitamin A (beta-carotene)	4677 IU	94%

Carrots are available year round in all grocery stores and they are CHEAP. Raw or cooked there is no excuse why anyone should ever suffer from chronic Vitamin A deficiency.[16][53]

CELERY (EXCELLENT "NET NEGATIVE CALORIE" FOOD) – I discuss the concept of "Net negative calorie" foods in the above entry on Lettuce) Basically, the more celery you eat, the better because each celery stalk costs you more calories than you get back out of it. Even if it does actually provide you with a handful of calories (and I do mean less than 10) snacking on celery rather than cupcakes, cookies, potato chips and dip, etc. can transform your daily caloric intake from MANY THOUSANDS of excess and harmful trash calories to practically NONE. But the benefits of celery are not limited to just being a dieter's best friend. Celery is loaded with a bunch of phytonutrients that are either unique to it (and its kin: rhubarb, fennel plant and a few others) or found in far higher amounts in it than any other readily available foods.

ORAC Score: 552 (raw)

1 OZ. CONTAINS:		%DV
Calories	4.5	<1%

From Carbohydrate	3.3	(1)
From Fat	0.4	(1)
From Protein	0.8(0.2g)	<1%
Saturated Fat	0g	0%
Cholesterol	0mg	0%
Phytosterols	1.7mg	(3)
Total Omega-3 fatty acids	0mg	(1)
Total Omega-6 fatty acids	22.1mg	(1)
Fiber	0.4g	2%
Water	26.7g (94% by weight)	(1)
Vitamin A (beta-carotene)	126 IU	3%
Vitamin K	8.2mcg	10%

Aside from being a very low calorie snack food, Celery contains APIOLE which was once used to treat menstrual problems and APIGENIN which shows promise in helping regenerate damaged brain cells, weakening cancerous cells (making them more susceptible to everything from chemotherapy to our own immune system response) and serves as a kidney tonic helping the kidneys detoxify and recover from damage. Although all of the research is in the preliminary stages, I believe that celery does have these amazing health benefits because I eat it regularly and my brain and kidneys still work despite everything I did to them when I was young and foolish. [51][54][55][56]

*BROCCOLI (#1 SOURCE OF CHROMIUM) – Chronic deficiency of chromium which is very difficult to find in sufficient quantities to satisfy our RDA requirements of it CAN and WILL lead to late onset (Type II) diabetes. We don't need much, but since almost no other food with the exception of grapes and their by-products (see the entry for Grapes and Raisins in the section on fruits) has chromium in better than trace amounts, broccoli is not just another superfood, it is a NECESSITY. For those who don't like it, that sounds like bad news, but you will have to try. I hate beef liver with a passion, but I have found a way to incorporate it into my daily eating regimen so I understand the dilemma. Personally I slather all unsavory foods in enough butter and garlic or Oil and Vinegar, or even homemade cheese sauce that they simply get lost underneath the spices and flavors of these garnishes which happen to be very healthy for you too.

ORAC Score: 2160 (boiled)

1 OZ. CONTAINS:		%DV
Calories	9.5	<1%
From Carbohydrate	6.7	(1)
From Fat	0.9	(1)
From Protein	1.9(0.8g)	2%

Saturated Fat	0g	0%
Cholesterol	0mg	0%
Phytosterols	0mg	(3)
Total Omega-3 fatty acids	5.9mg	(1)
Total Omega-6 fatty acids	4.8mg	(1)
Fiber (raw broccoli)	0.7g	3%
Water	25.0g (88% by weight)	(1)
Vitamin A (beta-carotene)	174 IU	3%
Vitamin C	25.0mg	42%
Vitamin K	28.4mcg	36%
Chromium	22mcg	18%

Slightly more than 5 oz. of Broccoli will provide 100%RDA of Chromium. One teaspoon of garlic also brings about 12%DV of Chromium. See Grapes and Raisins for the ONLY other significant source of this ESSENTIAL mineral.[57][58]

PLANT SUPERFOODS – THE LEGUMES

All legumes are by the strictest definition, SECONDARY foods. However, since they require far less cooking than most beans, we have to call them sort of "in-betweeners" and that makes them close enough that we can make an exception for them especially since they are LOADED with essential nutrients and some are the ONLY readily available sources of those nutrients for most people. But they are still SECONDARY foods which means that they should not be eaten daily unless the alternative is to go without the nutrient they are providing or to take MANUFACTURED pills. It is still highly preferable to eat some green peas as a side dish with dinner than to take a supplement containing CHEMICALS that were manufactured in Frankenstein's lab. All of the legumes are relatively fast growing plants and thus contain higher quantities of Molybdenum in them than most other foods as well.

***CHICK PEAS** (boiled, no salt, EXCELLENT SOURCE OF FOLATE, MANGANESE, & MOLYBDENUM) – If you are eating your seeds and nuts, then you know that you are already getting loads of Manganese, which means that Chick Peas could lead you to consuming drastic excesses if you eat them daily. If you have decided to pass on the seeds and nuts then you have a big problem – where will you get your Vitamin E? Folate is extremely difficult to get in sufficient quantities from most foods and even a cup of chick peas will not provide you with 100% RDA but it will provide you with about 70% which is a very good start to getting enough for the day. I included chick peas as a superfood because they are readily available year round in most grocery stores either dried and bagged or pre-cooked and canned. Just try to find "no salt" versions in LINED cans (have a layer of white latex to prevent metal ions from getting into the food which can and will cause METAL POISONING.) And chick peas can be used to make

hummus, which is one of the few dips or spreads that does NOT contain RAW EGGS which are TERRIBLE and must be avoided (that includes all products made from raw eggs including mayonnaise and most creamy salad dressings and dips.)
ORAC Score: 847 (raw)

1 OZ. CONTAINS:		%DV
Calories	45.9	2%
From Carbohydrate	31.2	(1)
From Fat	6.1	(1)
From Protein	8.6(2.5g)	5%
Saturated Fat	0.1g	0%
Cholesterol	0mg	0%
Phytosterols	0mg	(3)
Total Omega-3 fatty acids	12.0mg	(1)
Total Omega-6 fatty acids	312.0mg	(1)
Fiber	2.1g	9%
Water	16.9g (60% by weight)	(1)
Vitamin B9 (Folate)	48.2mcg	12%
Manganese	0.3mg	14%
Molybdenum	34mcg	46%

A FIVE oz. serving contains 45%DV Fiber, 230%DV Molybdenum, 60%DV Folate, and 70%DV Manganese. Chick peas are a superfood because they can be used to make hummus, a very healthy alternative dip or spread. Mayo and its kin (most creamy salad dressing and dips) are DETRIMENTAL to your health and should be ELIMINATED from your diet altogether. That megablast of Molybdenum is what truly makes Chick peas a superfood. Molybdenum is used to create Molybdenum Cofactor in the body (MOCO) and this is what facilitates our ability to turn raw sulfur compounds found in foods like garlic and onions, broccoli and cabbage, into useful compounds like some of the amino acids (which are used to construct all proteins in all cells in the human body) as well as much more interesting things like Vitamin B1 (Thiamine also contains a sulfur atom.) [28][37][59][60]
*LENTILS (boiled, no salt, EXCELLENT SOURCE OF FOLATE, FIBER & #1 SOURCE of MOLYBDENUM) – I am working on an upcoming volume that will start a series of Health Food Cookbooks and the legumes will get their fair share of recipes. For me, lentils are nearly impossible to cook correctly (I always end up under-cooking them or overcooking them) so keep an eye out for these volumes because lentils are highly preferable to chick peas for one reason: they are not overloaded with Manganese which in turn allows you to eat all of those wonderful seeds and nuts without worrying about overdoing it on Manganese.
ORAC Score: 7282 (Very Good)

1 OZ. CONTAINS:		%DV
Calories	32.5	2%
From Carbohydrate	22.8	(1)
From Fat	0.9	(1)
From Protein	8.8(2.5g)	5%
Saturated Fat	0g	0%
Cholesterol	0mg	0%
Phytosterols	0mg	(3)
Total Omega-3 fatty acids	10.4mg	(1)
Total Omega-6 fatty acids	38.4mg	(1)
Fiber	2.2g	9%
Water	19.5g (69% by weight)	(1)
Vitamin B9 (Folate)	50.7mcg	13%
Molybdenum	49mcg	65%

A FIVE oz. serving of lentils contains 45%DV Fiber, 325%DV Molybdenum, and 65%DV Folate. Lentils have a far lower amount of Manganese in them which makes them an excellent alternative to chick peas for those who have chosen to eat a lot of seeds and nuts which I highly recommend and they have the highest concentration of molybdenum of just about any food on Earth. Eating lentils just twice a week (5 oz. serving) is all you need in order to get plenty of this essential micronutrient.[30][37][59][61]

***GREEN PEAS** (boiled, drained, EXCELLENT SOURCE OF MOLYBDENUM, LOW CALORIE FOOD) – Green peas make the grade because they are available year round in all grocery stores either dried and bagged or boiled and canned. Just be sure to get the "No salt" version in LINED cans to avoid METAL POISONING. Green peas are tied with lentils as the #1 source of Molybdenum but are not a significant source of any other nutrients. They do have far fewer calories per ounce however, and for those who are eating plenty of seeds and nuts this makes them the better choice as your regular source of molybdenum.

ORAC Score: 120 to 300 (canned, cooked)

1 OZ. CONTAINS:		%DV
Calories	19.3	1%
From Carbohydrate	12.8	(1)
From Fat	1.6	(1)
From Protein	5.0(1.3g)	3%
Saturated Fat	0g	0%
Cholesterol	0mg	0%
Phytosterols	0mg	(3)
Total Omega-3 fatty acids	8.7mg	(1)
Total Omega-6 fatty acids	37.0mg	(1)

Fiber	1.4g	5%
Water	23.1g (81% by weight)	(1)
Molybdenum	49mcg	65%

A 5 oz. serving contains 25%DV Fiber and 325%DV Molybdenum. Green peas will have plenty of entries in the upcoming volumes on Healthy Recipes.[30][59][62]

***PEANUTS or PEANUT BUTTER** (smooth, avg. values) – Although unsalted dry roasted peanuts are a far healthier choice, the nutritional content of peanut butter is very close to them (identical if it is 100% natural with no additives and no salt) and this product is available in all stores throughout the year. Peanuts and peanut butter make the superfoods list because they are good source of Niacin, Vitamin E, Magnesium and Phosphorus. ORAC Score: 3432 (Good)

1 OZ. CONTAINS:		%DV
Calories	165	8%
From Carbohydrate	22.2	(1)
From Fat	118	(1)
From Protein	24.4(7.0g)	14%
Saturated Fat	2.9g	14%
Cholesterol	0mg	0%
Phytosterols	28.6mg	(3)
Total Omega-3 fatty acids	21.3mg	(1)
Total Omega-6 fatty acids	3861mg	(1)
Fiber	1.7g	7%
Water	0.5g (2% by weight)	(1)
Vitamin B3 (Niacin)	3.8mg	19%
Vitamin E	2.5mg	13%
Copper	0.1mg	7%
Magnesium	43.1mg	11%
Manganese	0.4mg	21%
Phosphorus	100mg	10%
Potassium	182mg	5%
Zinc	0.8mg	5%

A FIVE oz. serving of peanuts or peanut butter (and that is a LOT of peanut butter!) contains 95%DV Niacin, 65%DV Vitamin E, 55%DV Magnesium (a valuable source of this mineral) 105%DV Manganese, 35%DV Copper, 50%DV Phosphorus, 25%DV Potassium, and 25%DV Zinc. Most people do not track the minerals and peanut butter may be their ONLY SOURCE of Magnesium and Zinc but these come up way short even in five oz. ½ cup and a TRUCK LOAD of calories.[11][23][31][34][38][39][63]
Blackeye Peas: (17.2 cal/oz, High Fiber, Molybdenum)

PLANT FOODS – GRAINS

The grains are definitely SECONDARY FOODS on the "DO NOT EAT" list. These are basically 100% "undigestable" until they are cooked. Many are loaded with nutrients but on the whole they are simply not worth eating even to get those nutrients. Having said that, there are TWO grain products of interest: wheat germ (which is the pure nugget of nutrients within the wheat kernel) and whole wheat bread and the other grain food on the menu is old-fashioned oats. Both are high in molybdenum which is a critical micronutrient that we need on a daily basis.

***OATS** (Old-fashioned, EXCELLENT SOURCE OF FIBER, SAPONINS AND MOLYBDENUM) – Old-fashioned oatmeal is one of only two grain products that I highly recommend on a daily basis. It contains both fiber and saponins which are both highly beneficial to the digestive system; Fiber because it absorbs some cholesterol and thus blocks it from being absorbed by the intestines and the saponins which actually improve cellular membrane permeability (a fancy way of saying that they allow the intestinal walls to have a higher capacity to absorb other nutrients.) A bowl of oatmeal in the morning sets you up for better digestion for the rest of the day and gives you an opportunity to load it up with other excellent nutritious foods like raisins and walnuts too. ORAC Score: 1708

1 OZ. CONTAINS:		%DV
Calories	106	5%
From Carbohydrate	78.1	(1)
From Fat	15.3	(1)
From Protein	12.7(3.7g)	7%
Saturated Fat	0.3g	0%
Cholesterol	0mg	0%
Phytosterols	0mg	(3)
Total Omega-3 fatty acids	28mg	(1)
Total Omega-6 fatty acids	616mg	(1)
Fiber	2.8g	11%
Water	3.0g (10% by weight)	(1)
Vitamin B1 (Thiamine)	0.1mg	9%
Magnesium	38.6mg	10%
Manganese	1.0mg	51%
Molybdenum	33mcg	45%
Phosphorus	115mg	11%

Just 2 oz (about ½ cup) provides 22%DV Fiber, 18%DV Thiamine, 20%DV Magnesium, 100%DV Manganese (watch out for getting too much of this one daily), 90%DV Molybdenum (excellent readily available source of this trace essential nutrient), and 22%DV of

Phosphorus. While it is certainly not a superfood for providing partial amounts of most nutrients it qualifies because of the fiber, the molybdenum, and the saponins. Dress it up with a variety of goodies like raisins (high in Iron and the unique and powerful phytonutrients found in dark grapes) walnuts (excellent source of the plant Omega-3 – ALA) cinnamon (massive blast of powerful antioxidants) and wheat germ. [28][30][59][64][65]

***WHEAT GERM** (EXCELLENT SOURCE OF FOLATES AND MOLYBDENUM) – Wheat germ is the solid nugget of nutrients within the wheat kernel and is the most nutritious grain product you could ever eat. I put about 2.5 oz a day on my oatmeal for breakfast and although it has a LOT of manganese in it, it hasn't made me sick (yet!) Personally, I would recommend lower amounts and probably every other day just to play it safe with that mineral. Whole heat flour products are so much more nutritious than plain bleached white flour products precicely because the wheat germ nugget was kept in the making of the flour. Whole wheat flour products do have one item in them that is lacking in the wheat germ which makes them (things like 100% Whole Wheat Bread) and that is betaine which is an amino acid that has been linked to the reduction of homocysteine levels in the blood and therefore helps to control arterial plaque build up that can lead to heart attack and stroke. Don't hesitate to buy 100% Whole Wheat bread from now on but limit it to about two slices per day to avoid developing gluten intolerance.

ORAC Score: 380 (whole grain wheat)

1 OZ. CONTAINS:		%DV
Calories	101	5%
From Carbohydrate	54.7	(1)
From Fat	22.8	(1)
From Protein	23.3(6.5g)	13%
Saturated Fat	0.5g	2%
Cholesterol	0mg	0%
Phytosterols	0mg	(3)
Total Omega-3 fatty acids	202mg	(1)
Total Omega-6 fatty acids	1481mg	(1)
Fiber	3.7g	15%
Water	3.1g (81% by weight)	(1)
Vitamin B1 (Thiamine)	0.5mg	35%
Vitamin B6	0.4mg	18%
Folate	78.7mcg	20%
Molybdenum	49mcg	65%

Just THREE oz of Wheat germ contains 45%DV Fiber, 105%DV Thiamine, 54%DV Vitamin B6, 60%DV Folate and 195%DV

Molybdenum. Whole wheat grain products are high in these nutrients as well because the Wheat germ was kept in their production. Whole wheat grain products are also the #1 source of Betaine which reduces the quantity of homocysteine in the blood which in turn lowers cholesterol and reduces plaque build up in the arterial walls. Wheat as well as rye and barley also have alkyl-resorcinols in them which have been linked to the prevention of cancer.[30][33][36][37][59][66][67][68]

PLANT FOODS - FRUITS

This section holds many foods that you would not expect because you do not normally think of them as fruits. If we define "fruit" as the reproductive organ that holds the plant's seeds whether edible or not, then olives and tomatoes as well as cucumbers and all forms of squash are fruits by definition and they will be included in this section. The only thing that makes us call one such object like a grape a fruit and another like a cucumber a "vegetable" is really just their sugar content. And the cucurbits (cucumbers and their kin) are a vast family that does have some sugary fruit members including cantaloupes and watermelons (think about it, a water-melon even looks like an enormous cucumber! They might be very distantly related, but they are related.)

Even amongst the fruits there exist only a very small percentage of them that are edible to humans. Despite this fact there are literally many thousands of species of edible fruits on Earth. There are, for example, an estimated 160+ species of trees in the Annona genus alone and almost all of them produce edible fruit. And the only one that most folks have even heard of and likely never tried is the "Soursop." Don't be fooled by the name either, they are incredibly sweet and delicious too. The point is that there is no way I will be able to find the nutritional analysis of the vast majority of all edible fruits on Earth and I am confident that there are unusual fruits out there with incredible nutritional content, not just of the essential nutrients that we know about, but also for their specific and unique phytonutrients many of which have yet to even be identified by science like the constituents of the fruits of the trees of the Duguetia genus all of which are rare and endangered species found in the equatorial regions of the planet.

But the superfoods include those foods that are highly available to most people and are found at least part of the year in most well stocked grocery stores. So these common foods are the ones that will make this list, but in upcoming volumes I will cover many of these not-so-common fruits and other edible foods in the volumes on the "remedials" (and there will be many if I live long enough to get to them all.)

***BANANAS** (GOOD SOURCE OF POTASSIUM) – Everybody knows that bananas are high in potassium, but did you know that one large banana brings about 14% of your RDA of this critical mineral? That means you would have to eat SEVEN to EIGHT of

33

them a day to get all of the potassium you need on a daily basis. Potassium has the largest RDA of all essential nutrients; we need 3200mg per day which is a physically ENORMOUS amount. In the form of Potassium Chloride (once used as the salt substitute of choice in the early days of the medical industry's "No salt" crusade, but it tastes too metallic) that would be a full teaspoon of it. Needless to say, getting enough potassium in our daily diet is a real challenge and two bananas a day can go a long way toward reaching that goal.

ORAC Score: 795

1 OZ. CONTAINS:		%DV
Calories	24.9	1%
From Carbohydrate	23.1	(1)
From Fat	0.8	(1)
From Protein	1.0(0.3g)	1%
Saturated Fat	0g	14%
Cholesterol	0mg	0%
Phytosterols	4.5mg	(3)
Total Omega-3 fatty acids	7.6mg	(1)
Total Omega-6 fatty acids	12.9mg	(1)
Fiber	0.7g	3%
Water	21.0g (74% by weight)	(1)
Vitamin B6	0.1mg	5%
Vitamin C	2.4mg	4%
Potassium	100mg	3%
Manganese	0.1mg	4%

TEN ounces of bananas per day will bring 30%DV Potassium and 40%DV Manganese. It seems odd that bananas are a better source of Manganese than Potassium, but that is only because we need a HUGE amount of potassium and only a tiny amount of Manganese daily. In the "Top Recommended Superfoods" chapter I will cover ALL of the essential nutrients and how to get at least 100% RDA amounts of them on a daily basis from natural whole foods. By the way, bananas are a great source of CATECHINS which the body is always looking for and the liver "metabolizes" into different compounds that it releases into the blood that play key roles in human health. [28][39][69]

*CUCUMBERS (peeled, EXCELLENT "NET NEGATIVE CALORIE" FOOD) – I discuss the concept of "Net negative calorie" foods in the preceding entry on Lettuce and I have included the best of them in this list as superfoods because they are definitely the dieter's best friends and also make very healthy snacks and interesting additions to the daily salad which is the best way to get the dark leafy green vegetables into your diet.

ORAC Score: 140

1 OZ. CONTAINS:		%DV
Calories	3.4	<1%
From Carbohydrate	2.3	(1)
From Fat	0.4	(1)
From Protein	0.7(0.2g)	0%
Saturated Fat	0g	14%
Cholesterol	0mg	0%
Phytosterols	2.8mg	(3)
Total Omega-3 fatty acids	0.6mg	(1)
Total Omega-6 fatty acids	0.6mg	(1)
Fiber	0.2g	1%
Water	27.1g (95% by weight)	(1)
Vitamin K	2.0mcg	3%

Cucumbers have a few trace nutrients in them but they are not a significant source of anything. What makes them a superfood is that they actually have one of the lowest caloric values of any food. If there is a true "Net negative calorie" food on Earth, peeled cucumbers are it. Be sure to peel them because the skin is bad for you.[51][70]

GRAPEFRUIT (red, GREAT SOURCE OF VITAMIN C) – All citrus fruits are high in NATURAL FORM Vitamin C called L-ascorbic acid. There have been studies that show that artificial, concocted Vitamin C, which contains 50% each of the "left-handed" and "right-handed" molecules, is TOXIC. All plants ONLY make the correct form and it is FAR BETTER to get your Vitamin C from natural sources only. Grapefruit also contains an enzyme that facilitates the activation of processes in the body that will break down stored fat reserves. Grapefruits actually make the body burn fat and are a dieter's best friend. They are also one of the lowest calorie foods despite all of the fructose hiding beneath all of the citric acid that makes them sour. I try to have a whole grapefruit with no sugar added daily for breakfast and you should too. ORAC Score: 1548

1 OZ. CONTAINS:		%DV
Calories	11.8	1%
From Carbohydrate	10.7	(1)
From Fat	0.3	(1)
From Protein	0.7(0.2g)	0%
Saturated Fat	0g	14%
Cholesterol	0mg	0%
Phytosterols	0mg	(3)
Total Omega-3 fatty acids	0.6mg	(1)

Total Omega-6 fatty acids	0.6mg	(1)
Fiber	0.4g	2%
Water	24.7g (87% by weight)	(1)
Vitamin A (beta-carotene)	322 IU	6%
Vitamin C	8.7mg	15%

TEN ounces of grapefruit contains just 118 calories and provides 60%DV Vitamin A as beta-carotene (a safe antioxidant form) and 150% Vitamin C as the natural L-ascorbic acid form. [49][51][71]

***GRAPES and GRAPE JUICE** (Concord variety, EXCELLENT SOURCE OF CHROMIUM) –

ORAC Score: 2389 (Concord variety)

Grapes and their by-products including the juice, raisins and even wine contain hundreds of unique phytonutrients that have been linked to some of the most amazing health benefits of all foods including longevity (anti-aging,) combating cancer, and preventing Type II diabetes. They contain a whole host of antioxidants including Myricetin which is BOTH a powerful antioxidant bringing all of the health benefits of those AND an oxidant that shows amazing powers in fighting viruses, AT THE SAME TIME. Dark skinned varieties are best because these bring yet another set of powerful antioxidants known as anthocyanidins which are mostly found in foods colored blue to purple to black. 100% pure Concord grape juice has been shown in many studies to improve circulation by cleaning the blood vessels by removing plaque build-up on arterial walls and making them much more elastic which also improves blood pressure. You can't go wrong drinking about 24 ounces a day which will provide you with 100% RDA of Chromium, an essential mineral that most people don't get in their daily diets and are suffering from chronic deficiency of it which can and will lead to Type II diabetes. [13][57][72][73][74][75][76]

KIWI (EXCELLENT SOURCE OF VITAMIN C) – Most people don't realize that Kiwis have a higher concentration of Vitamin C than even the citrus fruits. Just two average sized Kiwis will satisfy your 100% RDA requirement for this important vitamin. We also realize that the 100% RDA amount is way short of what a person needs for OPTIMUM THRIVE-LEVEL health. [44][49][77]

1 OZ. CONTAINS:		%DV
Calories	17.1	<1%
From Carbohydrate	14.8	(1)
From Fat	1.2	(1)
From Protein	1.1(0.3g)	1%
Saturated Fat	0g	0%
Cholesterol	0mg	0%
Phytosterols	0mg	(3)
Total Omega-3 fatty acids	11.8mg	(1)

Total Omega-6 fatty acids	68.9mg	(1)
Fiber	0.8g	3%
Water	23.3g (82% by weight)	(1)
Vitamin C	26.0mg	43%
Vitamin K	11.3mcg	14%

ORAC Score: 862

***OLIVES and OLIVE OIL** (green or black, EXCELLENT SOURCE OF MANY UNIQUE PHYTONUTRIENTS) –

ORAC Score: 1010 (green) 370 (extra virgin olive oil)

Olives and Olive Oil are loaded with dozens upon dozens of unique phytonutrients only found in them. Research has only just begun into these compounds but many believe that they have enormous health benefits. While the fruit and the oil may not satisfy any of the essential nutrient requirements, because of all of these unique phytonutrients and the fact that oil and vinegar dressing should be the only one you use on your salad (by far the healthiest salad garnish) olives and olive oil are definitely superfoods.[78][79][80]

***TOMATOES** (primarily classic red, i.e. Beefsteak variety, EXCELLENT SOURCE OF LYCOPENE, and a NET NEGATIVE CALORIE FOOD) – I discuss "Net negative calorie" foods under the entry for Lettuce, but tomatoes do not make the superfoods list for that alone; they have one of the highest concentrations of, and are certainly the most available source of, Lycopene. Lycopene is one of the most powerful antioxidants known and our digestive tract knows all about it and absorbs it and sends it though the bloodstream throughout the body where it is involved in a whole litany of health benefits discussed in "The Truth About... Vol.4."

ORAC Score: 546

1 OZ. CONTAINS:		%DV
Calories	5.0	<1%
From Carbohydrate	4.0	(1)
From Fat	0.5	(1)
From Protein	0.6(0.2g)	0%
Saturated Fat	0g	14%
Cholesterol	0mg	0%
Phytosterols	2.0mg	(3)
Total Omega-3 fatty acids	0.8mg	(1)
Total Omega-6 fatty acids	22.1mg	(1)
Fiber	0.8g	3%
Water	26.5g (93% by weight)	(1)
Vitamin A (beta-carotene)	233 IU	5%
Vitamin C	2.6mg	6%

Tomatoes are an excellent low calorie zero cholesterol food that brings a lot of lycopene that has enormous health benefits. Cooking activates the lycopene making it even stronger. Canned (or prepackaged in jars) tomato sauce does not have the same power as cooking it fresh, so start making that homemade tomato sauce and throw in a bunch of super-powerful antioxidant-loaded spices too! [51][81][82]

HONORABLE MENTION: **Açai (ORAC Score 102700)**: this fruit comes from a species of palm tree that looks like a coconut tree and it is loaded with anthocyanidins (powerful antioxidants,) **Apples (ORAC Score 4275)**: loaded with antioxidants (only when eaten fresh; white apple flesh it good, ALL brown products are depleted) and many phytonutrients suspected of having enormous health benefits, **Apricots (ORAC Score 1110)**: these contain many interesting phytonutrients including catechins and should definitely be on the menu as well as the dried fruits (Prunes), **Avocados (ORAC Score 1922)**: high in Potassium, Vitamin K and useful phytonutrients including beta-sitosterol, **Black Raspberries (ORAC 19220), Blueberries**: much maligned as a thin skinned fruit (possibly contaminated with pesticides and fungicides) these are loaded with anthocyanidins (strong antioxidants,) **Cranberries (ORAC Score 9090)**: this tart fruit is loaded with anthocyanidins and other interesting phytonutrients and is very healthy for you (the juice is too,) **Gac** (Vietnamese fruit, #1 Source of Lycopene,) **Elderberries (ORAC 14697,) Mulberries (ORAC Score 6130)**: studies are showing that mulberries have many amazing health benefits, unfortunately they don't last long after being picked (due to their very high antioxidant content) so you might have to grow your own, **Passionfruit**: the studies are only just starting, but it looks like passionfruit may turn out to have extraordinary health benefits (can't find the fruit? The juice is good too,) **PECAN NUTS (ORAC 17940,) Pomegranates (ORAC Score 55520)**: While I find these impossible to eat (loaded with hard seeds) they contain several unique phytonutrients and studies are showing that they are incredibly powerful remedials for the human body and have the highest ORAC score of any fruit (fresh juice is just as good.) **Watermelon** (red flesh, high in Lycopene) [74][81][83][84]

PLANT SUPERFOODS - SPICES

The spices are truly amazing. They contain some of the most powerful biologically active phytonutrients found in any type of food and because many have been desiccated (dried and powdered) most of the water has been removed making them concentrates that are still "ready-to-eat." No one in their right mind is going to chew on straight powdered cloves, but you can put it right into your favorite stews, soups, etc. And because the spices are dehydrated concentrates they have astronomical ORAC Scores. Some of the highest scores belong to a handful of superfood vegetables and fruits that score between 7000 and

15000 but that's nothing compared to some of the spices on your cupboard shelf that score 100,000 to over 300,000! So if you have a spice sitting in your kitchen right now that has over 400 TIMES the antioxidant power of raw carrots, why not use it! Think about that for a moment; how many slices do you get out of a typical carrot when you chop it up? 20? One teaspoon of cloves (ORAC score: 290,000+) is about the size of one of those carrot slices and still has 20 TIMES the antioxidant power of the entire raw carrot. (It has the antioxidant power of the entire BAG of carrots!)

In this section I will forego the complete nutrient facts tables because we don't eat spices in sufficient quantity to fulfill any of the major nutrient requirements, but that doesn't mean they are any less significant especially when it comes to being the ONLY sources of a whole plethora of amazing phytonutrients that can definitely shore up your health.

CINNAMON (EXCELLENT SOURCE OF PHYTONUTRIENTS AND ANTIOXIDANTS) –

ORAC Score: 131420 (dried powder)

Cinnamon contains phytonutrients that assist the liver in blood sugar regulation and I can feel the difference (I have a strong tendency toward hypoglycemia and diabetes because everyone else in my family has these afflictions.) A daily dose of cinnamon can definitely help stave off these dreadful diseases and it provides a huge blast of antioxidants too. I dump a tablespoon of dried powder into my morning oatmeal every day.[85]

CLOVES (MANY UNIQUE PHYTONUTRIENTS AND TOP SOURCE OF ANTIOXIDANTS) –

ORAC Score: 290,283 (dried powder)

While there are a few foods with higher ORAC scores than ground cloves, they are not nearly as available to the average consumer as cloves. Any well stocked grocery store will have it in the spice aisle and it possesses tremendous health benefits.[86]

GARLIC (MANY UNIQUE PHYTONUTRIENTS including the GLUCOSINOLATES, EXCELLENT SOURCE OF CHROMIUM) –

ORAC Score: 6665 (dried powder) 5708 (fresh raw)

It's not just for keeping Vampires away, Garlic has been the subject of many studies throughout the years and its health benefits are legendary. Eating lots of garlic actually keeps mosquitoes from biting (although they will buzz you, maybe this is where the legend of keeping vampires away got started?) Garlic definitely helps lower cholesterol and also helps with blood sugar because it has a huge amount of chromium in it which is linked to proper insulin function. Garlic is also one of the best sources of glucosinolates, readers of "Vol. 4 – Antioxidants, Fiber and More" know that this means "the sulfur compounds." While there is no RDA for sulfur, all life on Earth needs it because it is found in several amino acids as well as Vitamin B1 – Thiamine and just one teaspoon of minced garlic contains 12% RDA of Chromium. I use it by the tablespoon in just about everything.[57][87][88]

OREGANO (EXCELLENT SOURCE OF CARVACROL AND ANTIOXIDANTS) –

ORAC Score: 175295 (dried) 13970 (fresh)

Carvacrol is a powerful antioxidant that has shown promise in current research as an anti-cancer agent (helps prevent and combat the disease.) Oregano lends a wonderful flavor to food and I use it, fresh and dried, in everything from my Oil and Vinegar salad dressing to soups and stews.[89][90]

ROSEMARY (EXCELLENT SOURCE OF CARNOSOL AND ANTIOXIDANTS) –

ORAC Score: 165280 (dried)

Carnosol is similar in molecular structure and function to Carvacrol (See Oregano) and as such it has shown promise in combating cancer. Rosemary has a strong pine-like aroma and flavor (from Betulinic acid, also under investigation for its suspected health benefits) and a lot of people may not like it in the amounts I use, but you should still try to sneak it into your soups and stews.[91][92][93]

SAGE (EXCELLENT SOURCE OF CARNOSOL, PERILLYL ALCOHOL AND ANTIOXIDANTS) –

ORAC Score: 119929 (dried powder)

Sage is definitely powerful medicine! Aside from its ORAC Score making it very beneficial to your overall health in being able to relieve oxidative stress in most organ systems in the body from your skin to your bones and everything in between, it also contains Carnosol and Perillyl alcohol both of which have shown evidence that they can combat cancer. This puts sage at the top of my list of spices and I use it liberally in just about everything I eat.[91][94][95]

TURMERIC (#1 SOURCE OF CURCUMIN AND ANTIOXIDANTS)

ORAC Score: 127068 (dried powder)

While most of the scientific community and big business would like to convince you that Curcumin has no effect – they are WRONG. Turmeric and its principle active phytonutrient, Curcumin, have too many medical experts supporting it as effective in the prevention and treatment of cancer. I try to get it into everything I cook and so should you.[96]

BLACK PEPPER (preferably ground fresh peppercorns, EXCELLENT SOURCE OF GLUCOSINOLATES and ANTIOXIDANTS) –

ORAC Score: 34053

Don't be shy with the black pepper! It has one of the highest ORAC Scores (high in antioxidants) of the regular spices that most people use. It also contains Piperine which has been shown to kill colon cancer cells and helps the absorption of all other nutrients in the digestive tract. It also contains Capsaicin, although not in the concentrations found in red hot peppers, which is also being investigated for its health benefits too.[97][98][99]

IODIZED SALT or SEA SALT (TOP AVAILABLE SOURCE OF IODINE) – Salt is also the most convenient source of both Sodium and Chlorine, both are ESSENTIAL nutrients that the body needs in large quantities daily. The problem is that Americans in particular are exposed to WAY TOO MUCH salt on a daily basis from fast foods to junk foods to canned foods. If you ELIMINATE ALL of that nonsense, then add 1 teaspoon of IODIZED or SEA SALT to your cooking to GUARANTEE coverage of your daily requirement of IODINE.[108]

HONORABLE MENTION: (High ORAC Scores): **Allspice** 100400, **Basil** 61063, **Cumin** (ground) 50372, **Curry powder** 48504, **Ginger** (ground) 39041, **Marjoram** 92310, **Nutmeg** 69640, **Parsley** 73670, **Peppermint** (dried) 160820, **Thyme** 157380.[83]

PLANT SUPERFOODS - OTHER

***BEETS** (CONTAIN A HOST OF UNIQUE PHYTONUTRIENTS and EXCELLENT SOURCE OF BETAINE) – As a child I ate almost every food my folks put in front of me and beets were NOT one of them. However, as an adult I have done my research and found that beets are loaded with a bunch of phytonutrients either unique to them or found in much larger quantities than any other source called the Betalains. There is a lot of research into these remarkable phytonutrients and the outlook is very promising too. Beets have the second highest concentration of betaine, an amino acid that helps control homocysteine levels in the blood which alleviates plaque build up that can lead to atherosclerosis and heart attack or stroke. The research has only just begun so we still do not know the full extent of the health benefits of beets, but that's no reason to wait; so eat your beets!

ORAC Score: 1776

1 OZ. CONTAINS:		%DV
Calories	8.7	1%
From Carbohydrate	7.6	(1)
From Fat	0.3	(1)
From Protein	0.7(0.3g)	1%
Saturated Fat	0g	14%
Cholesterol	0mg	0%
Phytosterols	0mg	(3)
Total Omega-3 fatty acids	1.1mg	(1)
Total Omega-6 fatty acids	12.6mg	(1)
Fiber	0.5g	2%
Water	25.5g (90% by weight)	(1)
Iron	0.5mg	3%
Betaine	71.5	(1)

Beets may not be loaded up with essential nutrients but the phytonutrients and the betaine make them worth adding to your weekly diet. They are also an excellent "Net negative calorie" food making them a dieter's best friend. A SIX ounce serving only brings about 50 calories. It is amazing that beets bring so much Betaine when they are mostly water. [51][66][100][101]

***DARK CHOCOLATE** (EXCELLENT SOURCE OF IRON, MAGNESIUM, CATECHINS AND ANTIOXIDANTS) – Most people think I am crazy when I bring up Dark Chocolate as a superfood when in fact it makes the Top Recommended Superfoods list with little doubt once you see why. Aside from clams (#1) Dark Chocolate is the next best source of Iron. It takes four ounces to deliver 100% RDA amount of Iron, but did you know that it takes almost a POUND of beef liver to deliver that much Iron? No one should eat a pound of beef liver a day because all of that cholesterol would set you up for a heart attack, but the dark chocolate has ZERO CHOLESTEROL. I am not describing CANDY BARS here either, but 100% PURE CACAO mass which you can find in your local grocery store as "Baker's Unsweetened Chocolate Bars." Just read the ingredients label and make that there is only ONE ingredient: Chocolate or Cacao. Pure dark chocolate is quite bitter so sweeten it by dipping it into pure raw bee honey which is also GOOD FOR YOUR HEALTH.

ORAC Score: 49944

1 OZ. CONTAINS:		%DV
Calories	140	7%
From Carbohydrate	11.1	(1)
From Fat	123	(1)
From Protein	6.6(3.6g)	7%
Saturated Fat	9.1g	45%
Cholesterol	0mg	0%
Phytosterols	0mg	(3)
Total Omega-3 fatty acids	32.8mg	(1)
Total Omega-6 fatty acids	402.0mg	(1)
Fiber	0.4g	2%
Water	24.7g (87% by weight)	(1)
Iron	4.9mg	27%
Magnesium	91.6mg	23%
Phosphorus	112mg	11%
Copper	0.9mg	45%
Manganese	1.2mg	58%

While 4 ounces of dark chocolate (100% pure cacao) will bring you 100% RDA of Iron and Magnesium and 44%DV Phosphorus, it will also bring you 560 calories,180%DV Copper and 232%DV

Manganese. I do not recommend exceeding the RDA of these two metals on a continual daily basis which means you will have to seek your Magnesium and Iron from other sources as well as chocolate. And by the way, Chocolate has one of the highest concentrations of antioxidants too! [13][18][23][28][38][102]
***SPIRULINA** (dried, EXCELLENT SOURCE OF IRON) – For those who hate chocolate and prefer the taste of blue-green algae, spirulina is the way to go (Huh?) It does have a strong taste and it does taste like blue-green algae to me, but it does have a number of amazing health benefits including the fact that it is loaded with both Iron and Vitamins B1 – Thiamine and B2 – Riboflavin which are otherwise hard to find in significant quantities in most foods. If you decide to try it, don't buy too much (Trust me.) No ORAC Score available.

1 OZ. CONTAINS:		%DV
Calories	81.2	4%
From Carbohydrate	23.8	(1)
From Fat	18.1	(1)
From Protein	39.3(16.1g)	32%
Saturated Fat	0.7g	4%
Cholesterol	0mg	0%
Phytosterols	0mg	(3)
Total Omega-3 fatty acids	230mg	(1)
Total Omega-6 fatty acids	351mg	(1)
Fiber	1.0g	4%
Water	24.7g (87% by weight)	(1)
Vitamin B1 (Thiamine)	0.7mg	44%
Vitamin B2 (Riboflavin)	1.0mg	60%
Vitamin B3 (Niacin)	3.6mg	18%
Pantothenic acid	1.0mg	10%
Iron	8.0mg	44%
Magnesium	54.6mg	14%
Copper	1.7mg	85%
Manganese	0.5mg	27%

A THREE oz. serving of Dried Spirulina contains 132%DV Thiamine, 180%DV Riboflavin, 54%DV Niacin, 30%DV Pantothenic acid, 132%DV Iron, 42%DV Magnesium, 255%DV Copper and 81%DV Manganese. Because of the high levels of copper I also recommend eating spirulina sparingly (two or three times a week and NOT overdoing copper and manganese on the other days.) [13][14][18][28][33][34][38][103]
***V-8 BRAND VEGETABLE JUICE, ORIGINAL LOW SODIUM** (TOP SOURCE OF POTASSIUM) – Reader's of "Vol. 3 – Minerals and the Other Essential Nutrients" know that Potassium can be

nearly impossible to get in 100% RDA amounts. Even bananas simply do not have enough in them. We need more Potassium than any other essential nutrient other than air, water, and calories; 3200mg daily. In the form of Potassium chloride that is a whole teaspoon. So much that even the popular "A to Z" supplements only provide a few percent at best because the pills aren't physically LARGE enough to bring you all that you need. And Potassium is critical, chronic deficiency can lead to high blood pressure and uncontrollable muscle twitches which are a symptom of sudden acute Potassium deficiency and there is ONE muscle in your body that better never get those twitches: your HEART. Sudden acute Potassium deficiency can definitely give you a heart attack and kill you out of the blue and it is nearly impossible to get from any source in significant quantities other than low sodium vegetable juices that maintain their salty flavors with a TRUCK LOAD of Potassium salts.

ORAC Score: about 550

EIGHT OZ. CONTAINS:		%DV
Calories	51	3%
From Carbohydrate	43.1	(1)
From Fat	0	(1)
From Protein	8.0(2.0g)	4%
Saturated Fat	0g	14%
Cholesterol	0mg	0%
Phytosterols	0mg	(3)
Total Omega-3 fatty acids	0mg	(1)
Total Omega-6 fatty acids	0mg	(1)
Fiber	1.9g	8%
Water	228g (94% by weight)	(1)
Vitamin A (beta-carotene)	2000 IU	40%
Vitamin C	71.9mg	120%
Potassium	819mg	23%

Campbell Soup Company's Low Sodium V-8 is an excellent zero fat and zero cholesterol low calorie drink loaded with Vitamin A, Vitamin C and Potassium. 24 oz per day will provide you with about 68%DV Potassium which is otherwise incredibly difficult to get in 100% RDA amounts on a daily basis. Add two large bananas and you have completed your requirement of potassium for the day.[39][104]

(1)   – No firm RDA established for this constituent in foods.

(2)   – Complete Protein contains all nine essential amino acids in sufficient quantities to meet the RDA requirements of them.[105]

(3)   – Phytosterols can help reduce cholesterol and include many compounds that may turn out to be important. (alpha-Tocopherol, a.k.a. Vitamin E is a phytosterol.)

In the preceding three books in the series I describe the entire pantheon of the 41 essential nutrients (and I know that there are many sources that list higher numbers of essential nutrients than 41; one source I found online was saying that there are 90 of them) including the horrific consequences of chronic deficiencies as well as the often amazing benefits of getting them in at least the 100% RDA amounts. But most people on a pure junkfood/fastfood diet don't go blind from a lack of Vitamin A, or die from beriberi or pellagra, so many people wonder if these essential nutrients are as essential as all of the experts claim.

 While we do need Vitamin A on a daily basis, it turns out that we don't actually need very much of it: 5000 IU (International Units) of either retinol (true animal Vitamin A) or beta-carotene (a plant source Vitamin A precursor that we can process into Vitamin A as needed) but 1 IU of retinol is 0.3 micrograms or 0.6 micrograms for beta-carotene. That's 150 micrograms or a little less than 1/6 of one milligram of retinol or 300 micrograms of beta-carotene or about 1/3 of a milligram. While carrots are certainly loaded up with beta-carotene, tomatoes and many other red, orange and yellow colored vegetables have some in them as well. And eggs have some retinol in them. The point is that while a person could go for decades on lower than recommended amounts of Vitamin A and not go blind, they are setting themselves up for cataracts, macular degeneration and a host of other vision problems later in life. And that's the real kicker about all of these nutrients: you might get away with a horrific diet for decades, but eventually the bill will come due and you will pay dearly for eating nothing but cancer-causing poisons deficient in most if not all of the essential nutrients that the body needs to maintain OPTIMUM THRIVE-LEVEL health.

 And there can be a significant difference between severe chronic deficiency versus mild chronic deficiency as well. With some essential nutrients, even mild chronic deficiency (getting at least some of the nutrient on a daily basis) can over time lead to a catastrophic consequence like a heart attack seemingly out of the blue, or cancer. In other cases, especially the B Vitamins, chronic mild deficiency could lead to premature aging and a host of psychological problems including irritability, depression, confusion and eventually memory loss as well as a noticeable decline in cognitive function: the inability to THINK, REASON, or SOLVE PROBLEMS.

 Chronic mild to severe deficiency in iodine can and will lead to reduced thyroid function or hypothyroidism which results in a lowered metabolism which in turn leads to the inability to warm up or to stay warm in a well air-conditioned building, and an increased tendency to want to stay inactive and of course obesity which aggravates the reduction in cardiovascular health and can lead to heart disease and ultimately kill the person decades ahead of their time. You will get no argument from me that Death is chasing after us all, but there is no reason and no excuse to go chasing after it.

This chapter is essentially a "reverse nutrient directory" of the superfoods listed in the preceding chapter. In this chapter you can look up a given nutrient like Vitamin A and see how much of each superfood it will take to get at least the 100% RDA amount. This list is LOADED with **HONORABLE MENTION** foods too.

THE NUTRIENTS AND THE FOODS THAT HAVE THEM

A, VITAMIN – See Retinol for animal sources and See Beta-carotene for plant sources.

ALKYLRESORCINOLS – WHEAT, **RYE** AND **BARLEY** (whole grain only) Linked to cancer prevention.[67]

ALPHA-LINOLEIC ACID (ALA, the plant Omega-3 Fatty Acid) – WALNUTS (2oz, 5200mg)[1][29]

ALPHA-TOCOPHEROL (Vitamin E) – ALMONDS (3oz, 100%DV), SUNFLOWER SEED KERNELS (3oz, 100%DV), PEANUTS (and Peanut butter, 5oz, 65%DV)[31][32][40][63]

ANTHOCYANIDINS – RED and PURPLE GRAPES, DARK RAISINS, MULBERRIES, BLUEBERRIES, CRANBERRIES, AÇAI, POMEGRANATE, RED DELICIOUS APPLE. These are very powerful antioxidants.[74]

ANTIOXIDANT – This is an enormous class of compounds and there are thousands of them and most plant foods contain them because the plants use them just like we do. Lucky for them, they can manufacture them for themselves while we have to chop them up and feast on them in order to get these vital nutrients. I have included the ORAC scores (Oxygen Radical Absorption Capacity) with each nutritional content table of every food so that you can see how they rate. The ORAC score described in detail in "Vol. 4 Antioxidants, Fiber, and More" can be treated as an arbitrary scale where 0 – 450 = Poor to Average, 450 – 1450 = Good, 1450 – 4500 = Very Good, 4500 – 15,000 = Excellent, and 15,000 – 50,000 = Outstanding, and 50,000+ = SUPER antioxidant food. But you cannot replace one low antioxidant food with one with a much higher score because different antioxidants play different roles in the body. While carrots stack up as barely "Good" on this scale, they contain beta-carotene as their primary antioxidant and this may be the only source of Vitamin A for many people. Use the ORAC scores to find SUPER antioxidant foods to ADD to your weekly diet.[75]

APIGENIN – CELERY. Linked to regeneration of brain tissue, attacks cancer cells, and relieves kidney stress and can support kidney regeneration.[55]

APIOLE – CELERY, PARSLEY. Was used in the past to treat menstrual problems and other female health issues including menopause.[54]

ASCORBIC ACID (Vitamin C) – KIWI (2, 100%DV), **GUAVA** (1, 100%DV), **CITRUS FRUITS** (varies), CABBAGE (4oz, 100%DV)[49][52][77]

ASTAXANTHIN – SALMON (Wild-caught,) **SHRIMP, CRAB, LOBSTER**. The highest concentrations are found in SALMON (the redder the better, it is what makes the flesh red) making SALMON one of the Top Recommended Superfoods.[8]

B1, VITAMIN – See Thiamine

B2, VITAMIN – See Riboflavin

B3, VITAMIN – See Niacin

B4, VITAMIN – Sometimes used to refer to Choline, but not universally accepted. See Choline.

B5, VITAMIN – See Pantothenic acid

B6, VITAMIN – See Pyridoxine

B7, VITAMIN – See Biotin

B9, VITAMIN – See Folate

B12, VITAMIN – See Methylcobalamin

BETA-CAROTENE – **WINTER/BUTTERNUT SQUASH** (2oz, 100%DV), **SWEET POTATO** (2oz., 100%DV), CARROTS (1 medium-sized, 200%DV)[16][53]

BETAINE – WHOLE WHEAT, BEETS. Reduces homocysteine levels in the blood which reduces plaque build up that leads to atherosclerosis, heart attack and stroke.[66][100]

BETALAINS – BEETS. Family of unique compounds found mostly in Beets that are currently being investigated.[100][101]

BETULINIC ACID – ROSEMARY. Shows some evidence that it might prevent cancer.[92][93]

BIOTIN (VITAMIN B7) – BEEF LIVER, EGGS, SALMON, **CAULIFLOWER**, WHEAT GERM, **WHOLE GRAIN BREAD** (all have over 100%DV for average adult)[6][7][68]

C, VITAMIN – See Ascorbic acid

CALCIUM – PARMESAN/ROMANO CHEESE (3oz, 100%DV), SWISS CHEESE (4.5oz, 100%DV), YOGURT (8oz, 50%DV), MILK (8oz, 30%DV) Everybody knows it is for the bones and teeth but it also contributes to blood vessel walls and even brain function. We need about 1000mg per day and it requires proper amounts of Magnesium, Vitamin K and Lysine so the body can actually use all of that Calcium.[21][22][24][25]

CAPSAICIN – **HOT PEPPERS**, BLACK PEPPERCORNS[99]

CATECHINS – GRAPES, RAISINS, GRAPE JUICE, WINE, APRICOTS, PRUNES, PRUNE JUICE, **PEACHES**, DARK CHOCOLATE, BANANAS, APPLES, **APPLE CIDER VINEGAR**. The digestive tract is always looking for these and absorbs them readily. The liver converts them into other compounds for use throughout the body.[84]

CHLOROPHYLLS – KALE, SPINACH, OTHER DARK LEAFY GREENS. Top liver detoxification nutrient.[46]

CHLORINE – IODIZED or SEA SALT (1tsp, 100%DV). Needed for some electrolytic functions (moving electrons in the nerves and the creation of hydrochloric acid in the stomach.

CHOLECALCIFEROL (Vitamin D3) – SUNLIGHT (2x20min exposures to face and arms, 100%DV) COD LIVER OIL (1Tbsp, >100%DV), SALMON (6 oz, 50%DV), MILK (8oz, 31%DV) Do not neglect this critical vitamin and stick to sources of the D3 form only. [6][26][27]

CHOLINE – BEEF LIVER (3oz. 50%DV), SALMON (6 oz, 50%DV), EGGS (1 large, 27%DV), PEANUTS (and Peanut butter, 5oz, 16%) This is a very difficult nutrient to get in 100% RDA amounts daily because we need a large amount of it. The good news is that it is present in most foods because it is the precursor to most of the other B vitamins. [6][17][19]

CHROMIUM – BROCCOLI (5oz, 100%DV), GRAPE JUICE (100% PURE CONCORD, 24oz, 100%DV), GARLIC (1tsp, 12%DV) [57][58][76][88]

COMPLETE PROTEIN – about 4 to 6oz any ANIMAL MEAT. Any animal meat brings Complete Protein which includes all nine essential amino acids: Isoleucine, Histidine, Leucine, Lysine, Methionine, Phenylalanine, Threonine, Tryptophan, and Valine.[105]

COPPER – Many superfoods bring copper and some in excessive quantities. Try not to exceed the 100%RDA of copper as much as you can because in extremely excessive amounts day after day it can become TOXIC.[18]

CURCUMIN – TURMERIC. Linked to cancer prevention and treatment.[96]

D, VITAMIN – See Cholecalciferol

DHA (DOCOSAHEXAENOIC ACID, always found together with EPA, the animal Omega-3's) –MACKEREL, SALMON, SARDINES, TUNA[1][2][3][6][9]

E, VITAMIN – See alpha-Tocopherol

EPA (EICOSAPENTAENOIC ACID) – See DHA.

FLAVONOIDS – Large group of compounds found in most plants. A healthy diet consisting of mostly natural whole foods and about 90% plants will include plenty of flavonoids.[106]

FOLATE – WHEAT GERM (2.3oz, 100%DV), CHICKPEAS (8oz, 100%DV), LENTILS (8oz, 90%DV), BEEF LIVER (3oz, 50%DV) [19][37][68][60][61]

GINGEROL – GINGER ROOT. Ginger root and its many unique compounds are currently under investigation for their long list of legendary health benefits.[107]

GLUCOSINOLATES – GARLIC, **ONION, CHIVE, SHALLOTS**, BROCCOLI, CAULIFLOWER, CABBAGE. The sulfur containing compounds are myriad and many are currently under investigation for a wide range of potential health benefits.[87]

HISTIDINE – One of the essential amino acids. See Complete Protein

IODINE – IODIZED SALT (1/2tsp, 100%DV), SEA SALT (1/2tsp, 100%DV), **KELP** (amounts vary), ORGANIC YOGURT (amounts vary). **COD** (Wild-caught, 3oz, 66%DV), EGGS (1 large, 16%DV) As long as you have dropped all of the fast food/junk food and packaged and processed and canned foods laced with POOR QUALITY salt without IODINE in it, you can now go back to consuming about 1 teaspoon of IODIZED SALT per day. SEA SALT is said to contain a better form and either salt is the easiest way to get Iodine.[108]

IRON – CLAMS (2.5oz, 100%DV), SPIRULINA (Dried, 3oz, >100%DV), DARK CHOCOLATE (4oz, 100%DV), BEEF LIVER (3oz, 25%DV) The World Health Organization estimates that 80% of the World's population is suffering from chronic iron deficiency. Very few foods have enough in them to meet our 100% RDA requirements of this critical mineral. Be sure you get enough on a daily basis. Two of the craziest sounding foods have enough: clams and dark chocolate.[12][13][19][102][103]

ISOLEUCINE – One of the essential amino acids. See Complete Protein

K, VITAMIN – See Phylloquinone

LEUCINE – One of the essential amino acids. See Complete Protein

LUTEIN – See Zeaxanthin

LYCOPENE – TOMATOES (Best source) GAC (Vietnamese fruit, #1 Source) WATERMELON (the redder; the better) Lycopene is a powerful antioxidant with of VERIFIED health benefits from years of clinical trials. [81]

LYSINE – One of the essential amino acids. See Complete Protein and usually deficient in plant protein.

MAGNESIUM – DARK CHOCOLATE (Baker's unsweetened, 4oz, 100%DV), ALMONDS (3oz, 60%DV), SUNFLOWER SEED KERNELS (5oz, 45%DV), PUMPKIN SEEDS (3oz, 54%DV), BRAZIL NUTS (2oz, 52%DV), PEANUTS (and peanut butter, 5oz, 55%DV), SPIRULINA (Dried, 3oz, 42%DV) Getting enough Magnesium in your diet can be a real challenge but we do need a LOT of it so you must pay attention to it and all of the minerals which are categorically difficult to get in 100% RDA amounts on a daily basis.[32][38][40][41][42][63][103]

MANGANESE – Many superfoods listed in this book are LOADED with Manganese and if you are switching to them you will almost certainly get your fill. Extreme excesses of Manganese (and MOST of the other minerals as well) can be TOXIC. So be careful of the foods you choose and try to stay at or near

100% RDA amounts and do not drastically exceed them day after day.[28]

METHIONINE – One of the essential amino acids. See Complete Protein and usually deficient in plant protein.

METHYLCOBALAMIN (Vitamin B12) – CLAMS (1oz, 461%DV), BEEF LIVER (1oz, 277%DV), SARDINES (2.5oz, 100%DV)[9][12][19]

MOLYBDENUM – WHEAT GERM, CHICKPEAS, GREEN PEAS, LENTILS. Eating any of these foods on a regular basis will ensure that you are getting plenty of Molybdenum. Like all of the metallic minerals, be sure that you do not exceed the 100% RDA amount by drastic amounts over a long period of time because it could become TOXIC.[59]

MYRICETIN – GRAPES, GRAPE JUICE, RAISINS, WINE [73]

NET NEGATIVE CALORIE FOODS – CUCUMBER, TOMATO, **ONION**, LETTUCE, CELERY, BEETS, GRAPEFRUIT, GREEN PEAS, BROCCOLI, **CAULIFLOWER**, CARROTS, CABBAGE, KALE, SPINACH (and ALL OTHER DARK LEAFY GREENS) See the entry on LETTUCE for more details. [51]

NIACIN – PEANUTS (and Peanut butter, 5oz, 100%DV), SUNFLOWER SEED KERNELS (5oz, 50%DV), SPIRULINA (Dried, 3oz, 50%DV), BEEF LIVER (3oz. 50%DV), TURKEY (5oz, 25%DV) Niacin is difficult to get in 100%RDA amounts from natural whole foods without committing to foods high in calories (the peanuts and the sunflower seed kernels are loaded with polyunsaturated fats.) However, it is far too important to ignore. [20][34][63][40][103]

OMEGA-3 FATTY ACIDS – See alpha-Linoleic acid (ALA) for the plant Omega-3 and DHA (Docosahexaenoic acid) for the animal Omega-3's You cannot completely depend on the plant Omega-3 (ALA) and you MUST get some animal Omega-3's into your daily diet.[1]

OMEGA-6 FATTY ACIDS – VEGETABLE OILS (Natural, not refined or processed like store bought oils) Most NUTS. The Omega-6 fatty acids are good for you but not in extreme excesses over the Omega-3's. Most research indicates that you should get no more than 3 TIMES as much Omega-6's as Omega-3's and that can be a challenge.[109]

ORGANIC ACIDS – Most plants particularly FRUITS from AÇAI to ZUCCHINI. While the combinations of these and flavonoids create the flavor of the food, they have a wide range of potential health benefits and most are currently being investigated.

PANTOTHENIC ACID (Vitamin B5) – SUNFLOWER SEED KERNELS (5oz, 100%DV), **CHICKEN LIVER** (Organic, 4oz, 100%DV) Pantothenic acid is found in almost all natural whole foods but in low quantities. Make it a point to look up this

Vitamin and make sure you are getting 100%DV on a regular basis.[35][40]

PHENYLALANINE – One of the essential amino acids. See Complete Protein

PHENYLETHANOIDS – OLIVES, OLIVE OIL. A small group of phytonutrients almost exclusive to Olives and Olive oil that are currently being researched for their suspected health benefits. Olive oil and vinegar should be the ONLY salad dressing you ever use.[78]

PHOSPHORUS – Most foods contain Phosphorus, these are the best: SUNFLOWER SEED KERNELS (3oz, 100%DV), PEANUTS (and Peanut butter, 5oz, 50%DV), DARK CHOCOLATE (Baker's unsweetened, 4oz, 44%DV), PISTACHIOS (3oz, 42%DV), BRAZIL NUTS (2oz, 40%DV), SWISS CHEESE (5oz, 80%DV), PARMESAN/ROMANO CHEESE (3 oz, 60%DV) MILK (8oz, about 25%DV) [22][23][24][40][42][43][63][102]

PHYLLOQUINONE (VITAMIN K1) – KALE, SPINACH, OTHER DARK LEAFY GREENS. [44]

PHYTOESTROGENS – Traces are found in many plant foods and are considered beneficial but in extreme excess like in SOY BEANS and their endless CHEAP GARBAGE FILLER BY-PRODUCTS they are considered potentially TOXIC which is why ALL SOY should be eliminated from your diet. [110]

POTASSIUM – V-8 BRAND LOW SODIUM VEGETABLE JUICE (8oz, 23%DV), BANANAS (2 large, 30%DV) Getting enough of this critical mineral is hard to do because we need a HUGE amount of it (3200mg) on a daily basis. Even supplements can't help because they would have to be the size of a quarter to hold that much potassium! Between the Low Sodium V-8 and the bananas you can get it done. Chronic Potassium deficiency COULD lead to ACUTE Potassium deficiency which can cause a HEART ATTACK out of nowhere. Chronic Potassium deficiency, I believe, is the #1 cause of HIGH BLOOD PRESSURE today.[39][69][104]

PYRIDOXINE (Vitamin B6) – TURKEY (6oz, 100%DV), TUNA (5oz, 50%DV), PISTACHIOS (5oz, 90%DV) [3][20][36][43]

RESVERATROL – GRAPES, GRAPE JUICE, RAISINS, WINE. Linked to longevity and anti-aging effects.[72][76]

RETINOL (animal source Vitamin A) – COD LIVER OIL (1Tbsp, >100%DV), BEEF LIVER (1oz, 95%DV) Many health professionals advise true animal source Vitamin A should be included in your regular diet as well as Beta-carotene (the plant source.) Whole fish like sardines, herring, smelts, and anchovies also bring some animal source Vitamin A. [16][19][27]

RIBOFLAVIN (Vitamin B2) – BEEF LIVER (3oz, >100%DV), LAMB (3oz, >100%DV), MILK (8oz, 26%DV), EGG (1 large,

13%DV) Without beef liver or lamb meat, Riboflavin is hard to get in 100%DV amounts on a daily basis. You should endeavor to look it up and get as much as you can. Two 8oz glasses of milk and 3 eggs will get you a long way, but that brings a lot of saturated fat and cholesterol (not that the liver and lamb are that much better!) [14][15][19]

SAPONINS – OATS [64][65]

SELENIUM – BRAZIL NUTS (Just 2 nuts, 100%DV), SUNFLOWER SEEDS KERNELS (3oz, 100%DV) and MOST FISH have plenty. [5][40][42]

SODIUM – IODIZED or SEA SALT. You still need 2900mg of Sodium per day. 1 teaspoon of IODIZED SALT daily gives you all of the Sodium, Chlorine and Iodine you need.[111]

SULFUR – GARLIC, **ONIONS**, BROCCOLI, CABBAGE, **CAULIFLOWER**, BLACK PEPPER, **CHIVES, SHALLOTS**, EGGS, FISH. All of these foods are high in sulfur compounds which are excellent for your health, just be sure to get some Molybdenum so that your body can UTILIZE all of that sulfur. [59][87][88][98]

THIAMINE (Vitamin B1) – SUNFLOWER SEED KERNELS (3oz, 100%DV), WHEAT GERM (3oz, 100%DV), SPIRULINA (Dried, 3oz, 100%DV), PISTACHIOS (3.5oz, 50%DV) [33][40][43][68][103]

THREONINE – One of the essential amino acids. See Complete Protein

TRYPTOPHAN – One of the essential amino acids. See Complete Protein and the entry on TURKEY.

VALINE – One of the essential amino acids. See Complete Protein

ZEAXANTHIN (and LUTEIN are found together) – KALE [47][48]

ZINC – OYSTERS (wild, 1oz, 170%DV), LAMB (5oz, 75%DV), SUNFLOWER SEED KERNELS (5oz, 50%DV), PUMPKIN SEEDS (3oz, 57%DV), PEANUTS (and Peanut butter, 5oz, 25%DV), SWISS CHEESE (5oz, 40%DV), PARMESAN or ROMANO CHEESE (3oz, 15%DV), CLAMS (3oz, 15%DV) Other than oysters, no single superfood can provide your 100% RDA of this critical nutrient involved in many enzymes within all of the cells in your body. Be sure to piece it together and make sure you get at least the 100% RDA amount daily. [10][11][12][15][22][24][40][41][63]

BE CONSISTENT

This means sticking with the plan for the rest of your longer, healthier and happier life, AND to get ALL of the ESSENTIAL NUTRIENTS in 100% RDA amounts. This will ensure that the body can properly utilize them all because most of these nutrients depend on others for proper absorption and usage throughout the body. Stay the course for the long haul until it becomes second nature to you and do not scrimp on any single nutrient.

In this chapter I will give you the "short version" of the superfoods lists like I did in the preceding three books. With this group of superfoods you can get ALL 41 ESSENTIAL NUTRIENTS quickly and easily on a daily basis. Certain nutrients like Potassium are extremely difficult to get even in the FDA's 100% RDA amount because it happens to be HUGE; so large that even foods with relatively high concentrations of it like bananas and avocados are still not good enough unless you eat far more than is practical So this list is basically worth the price of the book because with it you can make sure that you are getting EVERYTHING and in sufficient quantities to maintain OPTIMUM THRIVE-LEVEL health. In addition to the recognized 41 essential nutrients I have also included many other superfoods either because of their powerful array of specific phytonutrients or because of their incredibly high ORAC (Oxygen Radical Absorption Capacity) scores meaning that they are loaded with antioxidants.

ALMONDS (dry roasted, no salt, 3oz.) – 39% FIBER, 108% VITAMIN E, 42% RIBOFLAVIN, 48% COPPER, 60% MAGNESIUM, 111% MANGANESE, 42% PHOSPHORUS. [32]

ATLANTIC MACKEREL (5oz.) – 50% COMPLETE PROTEIN, 3,500mg DHA/EPA OMEGA-3 FATTY ACIDS,125% VITAMIN D3, 65% NIACIN, 205% VITAMIN B12, 90% SELENIUM. [2]

BANANAS (raw, 2 large fruits) – 30% POTASSIUM, 40%DV MANGANESE. [69]

BEEF LIVER (3oz.) – >100% RIBOFLAVIN, >100% VITAMIN A (as RETINOL,) 50% NIACIN, 825% VITAMIN B12, 25% IRON, 50% FOLATE, 50% CHOLINE, >100% BIOTIN, 33% COMPLETE PROTEIN. [19]

BEETS – BETALAINS, LOW CAL./ZERO CHOLESTEROL.[100]

BRAZIL NUTS (dry roasted, no salt, 2 nuts) – >100% SELENIUM. (Have a very high amount of Omega-6 fatty acids and you should not eat a lot of them on a daily basis.) [42]

BROCCOLI (raw or cooked, 5oz,) – 90% CHROMIUM, CHLOROPHYLL, and LOW CAL/ZERO CHOLESTEROL.[58]

CABBAGE (raw, 4oz.) – 100% VITAMIN C, 16% FOLATE, CHLOROPHYLL, and LOW CAL/ZERO CHOLESTEROL.[52]

CARROTS (raw, 1oz.) – 94% VITAMIN A (AS BETA-CAROTENE), and LOW CAL/ZERO CHOLESTEROL.[53]

CELERY (raw) – APIOLE, APIGENIN, LOW CAL./ZERO CHOLESTEROL.[54][55][56]

CHEESE, PAREMSAN or ROMANO (3oz.) – 60% COMPLETE PROTEIN,100% CALCIUM, 57% PHOSPHORUS, 27%DV SELENIUM, 15% ZINC.[22]

CHEESE, SWISS (unprocessed, 3oz.) – 45% COMPLETE PROTEIN, 48% VITAMIN B12, 66% CALCIUM, 48%

PHOSPHORUS, 21% SELENIUM, 18% ZINC.[24]

CHICKPEAS (canned, no salt, 5oz.) – 45% FIBER, 230% MOLYBDENUM, 60% FOLATE, 70% MANGANESE.[60]

COD LIVER OIL (1 Tablespoon) – 100% Vitamin A as Retinol, 150% Vitamin D as Cholecalciferol, 2664mg Omega-3 Fatty Acids as DHA and EPA.[27]

CLAMS (canned, wild, 3oz.) – 42% COMPLETE PROTEIN, 1380% VITAMIN B12, 30% COPPER, 130% IRON, 42% MANGANESE, 27% PHOSPHORUS, 15% POTASSIUM, 57% SELENIUM, 15% ZINC.[12]

CUCUMBERS (peeled) – LOW CAL./ZERO CHOLESTEROL.[70]

DARK CHOCOLATE (100% Pure cacao, Baker's Unsweetened, 4oz.) – 100% IRON, 100% MAGNESIUM, 180% COPPER, 44% PHOSPHORUS, 232% MANGANESE. ORAC: 49944 [102]

GRAPEFRUIT (red, 10oz.) – 150% VITAMIN C, 60% VITAMIN A, LOW CAL/ZERO CHOLESTEROL.[71]

GRAPE JUICE (100% Pure, Concord variety, 24oz.) – 100% CHROMIUM, ANTHOCYANIDINS, RESVERATROL, MYRICETIN, QUERCITIN, ETC.[57][72][73][74][76]

GREEN PEAS (boiled, no salt, 5oz.) – 325% MOLYBDENUM, 25% FIBER, LOW CAL./ZERO CHOLESTEROL.[59][62]

KALE (raw, 1oz.) – 86% VITAMIN A (AS BETA-CAROTENE), 56% VITAMIN C, 286% VITAMIIN K, 11% MANGANESE, CHLOROPHYLL, ZEAXANTHIN, LUTEIN, and LOW CAL./ZERO CHOLESTEROL.[47][48]

LAMB (5oz.) – 50% COMPLETE PROTEIN, 380% RIBOFLAVIN, 75% VITAMIN B12, 40% SELENIUM, 75% ZINC.[15]

LENTILS (boiled, no salt, 5oz.) – 45% FIBER, 65% FOLATE, 325% MOLYBDENUM.[61]

OATS (Old-fashioned oatmeal, 2oz.) – 22% FIBER, 18% THIAMINE, 20% MAGNESIUM, 100% MANGANESE, 90%DV MOLYBDENUM, 22% PHOSPHORUS, SAPONINS.[64][65]

OLIVES and OLIVE OIL – PHENYLETHANOIDS, OLEANOLIC ACID, ETC.[78][79][80]

OYSTERS (eastern, wild, canned, 1oz.) – 170% ZINC, 89% VITAMIN B12, 62% COPPER, 14% SELENIUM.[10]

PEANUTS (or Peanut butter, 5oz.) – 95% NIACIN, 65% VITAMIN E, 55% MAGNESIUM, 105% MANGANESE, 35% COPPER, 50% PHOSPHORUS, 25% POTASSIUM, 25% ZINC.[63]

PISTACHIOS (dry roasted, no salt, 3oz.) – 48% THIAMINE, 54% VITAMIN B6, 57% COPPER, 18% MAGNESIUM, 54% MANGANESE, 42% PHOSPHORUS, 18% POTASSIUM.[43]

POMEGRANATE (raw, fresh juice) – SEVERAL UNIQUE PHYTONUTRIENTS and ORAC Score: 55520 [112]

PUMPKIN SEEDS (whole, dry roasted, no salt, 3oz.) – 54% MAGNESIUM, 30% COPPER, 21% POTASSIUM, 21% MANGANESE, 57% ZINC.[41]

SALMON (Wild-caught, 5oz.) – 60% COMPLETE PROTEIN, 1,580mg DHA/EPA OMEGA-3 FATTY ACIDS, 55% NIACIN, 47% PANTOTHENIC ACID, 7.5MG BIOTIN (1000%DV FOR ADULTS,) 180% VITAMIN B12, 185% VITAMIN D3, 60% SELENIUM, PLUS ASTAXANTHIN.[6]

SARDINES (5oz.) – 70% COMPLETE PROTEIN, 2070MG OF DHA/EPA OMEGA-3, 210% VITAMIN B12, 95% VITAMIN D3, 55% CALCIUM 70% PHOSPHORUS, 105% SELENIUM.[9]

SPINACH (raw, 1oz.) – 53% VITAMIN A (AS BETA-CAROTENE), 169% VITAMIN K, 13% MANGANESE, CHLOROPHYLL, and LOW CAL./ZERO CHOLESTEROL.[45][46]

SPIRULINA (Dried, 3oz.) – 132% THIAMINE, 180% RIBOFLAVIN, 54% NIACIN, 30% PANTOTHENIC ACID, 132% IRON, 42% MAGNESIUM, 255% COPPER 81% MANGANESE.[103]

SUNFLOWER SEED KERNELS (3oz.) – 100% THIAMINE, 60% PANTOTHENIC ACID, 100% VITAMIN E, 100% PHOSPHORUS, 100% SELENIUM.[40]

TOMATOES (red raw or cooked) – LYCOPENE.[81][82]

TUNA (light, chunk, canned in water, 5oz.) – 70% COMPLETE PROTEIN, 400mg DHA/EPA OMEGA-3 FATTY ACIDS, 95% NIACIN, 50% VITAMIN B6, 70% VITAMIN B12, 160% SELENIUM.[3]

WALNUTS (English, 2oz.) – 5084mg ALA OMEGA-3 FATTY ACID, 44% COPPER, 96% MANGANESE.[1][29]

WHEAT GERM (crude or roasted, 3oz) – 45% FIBER, 105% THIAMINE, 54% VITAMIN B6, 60% FOLATE AND 195% MOLYBDENUM.[68]

V-8 ORIGINAL, LOW SODIUM (24oz.) – 68% POTASSIUM[104]

SPICE RACK (Top Choices) – **BLACK PEPPER** (preferably ground fresh peppercorns): PIPERINE (promotes absorption of all other nutrients in the digestive tract), ORAC Score: 34053, **CINNAMON**: ORAC Score: 131420, **CLOVES**: ORAC Score: 290,283, **GARLIC**: CHROMIUM, ORAC Score: 6665 (dried powder) 5708 (fresh raw,) **OREGANO**: CARVACROL, ORAC Score: 175295 (dried) 13970 (fresh,) **ROSEMARY**: CARNOSOL, BETULINIC ACID, ORAC Score: 165280 (dried,) **SAGE**: CARNOSOL, PERILLYL ALCOHOL, ORAC Score: 119929 (dried powder,) **TURMERIC**: CURCUMIN, ORAC Score: 127068 (dried powder) Most dried powdered spices are loaded with antioxidants **IODIZED or SEA SALT**: (BEST SOURCE OF IODINE) While this list includes some of the best; cilantro, basil, cumin, etc. are all good choices and are loaded with antioxidants and powerful phytonutrients as well.[83]

Back when the FDA made it law that all packaged foods had to carry a nutrition label, that label was far more extensive than the one they require nowadays. Most food manufacturers complained that the label was too large and therefore costly to print on their labeling especially for small items like candy wrappers, but the TRUTH ABOUT that was that they didn't want the public to see rows and columns of ZEROS – that their food was about as nutritious as boiled sawdust and contained almost no vitamins or minerals and was loaded with tons of trash calories in the forms of saturated fats, trans fats, processed sugars and cholesterol.

So the FDA caved in to the demands of the greedy billionaire monsters and now only requires a smaller "more concise" nutrient label on packaged foods as a bare minimum requirement to comply with the law. And this label really only brings two useful pieces of information now: 1) How many calories are in a single serving and 2) What form of calories they are. What is now lacking is the complete listing of the vitamins and minerals and all that is left on this new abbreviated nutrition label is Vitamin A, Vitamin C, Calcium and Iron. There is no question that these four are indeed important and as a matter of fact most people do not get nearly enough of either calcium or iron on a daily basis and chronic deficiency of either (and likely both) can lead to terrible consequences like disease and dying before your time.

However, all of the other vitamins, minerals and essential nutrients are just as important and chronic deficiencies in them can be just as bad (disease and death) but now we can't check the labels to see if the food is bringing enough things like Vitamin B5 – Pantothenic acid, or Chromium. Some nutrition labels will embellish them and list extra nutrients if the food has a good amount of them in it, so we can take away from this: if the nutrient is not in the nutrient label listing, then it has little to none in it

I have chosen as our typical sample nutrition label, the one included on the side of a typical box of "Macaroni and Cheese." This is a rather dreadful product for a number of reasons including the actual ingredients. I will skip that horror show here, but I do cover how to read ingredients labels in "The Truth About… Vol. 4 – Antioxidants, Fiber and More." Suffice it to say that it is loaded with chemicals and crud like processed wheat flour as well as that ubiquitous and apparently unstoppable bane: SOYBEAN by-products which are nothing more than CHEAP GARBAGE FILLERS. It takes up space and has weight and it is cheap which is why just about all packaged foods now have SOY in them, and many studies are now showing that this food is BAD FOR HUMAN CONSUMPTION; in other words, it is TOXIC. I bet the people who wrote and produced the movie "Soylent Green" had no idea how prophetic it would turn out to be. (Thankfully, the manufacturers of our foods are not cooking PEOPLE into little green squares yet!)

THE TYPICAL NUTRITION LABEL

The formats can be different and the one on the side of the slender box of "mac and cheese" that I am using is laid out differently than the way I shall present it here, but they all say the same things.

Nutrition Facts		
Serving Size 2.5oz (70g/about 1/3 box)		
Makes about 1 cup		
Servings per Container about 3		
Amount per Serving	**Mix**	**Prepared**
Calories	250	400
Calories from Fat	10	150
% Daily Value**		
Total Fat 1g*	**2%**	**26%**
Saturated Fat 0g	**0%**	**15%**
Trans Fat 0g		
Cholesterol 0mg	**0%**	**0%**
Sodium 580mg	**24%**	**31%**
Potassium 160mg	**5%**	**5%**
Total Carbohydrate 52g	**17%**	**18%**
Dietary Fiber 2g	**8%**	**8%**
Sugars 2g		
Protein 8g		
Vitamin A	0%	15%
Vitamin C	0%	0%
Calcium	2%	4%
Iron	10%	10%
Folic Acid	35%	35%

*Amount in mix. Prepared contributes an additional 150 calories (140 Calories from fat), 16g Total Fat (3g Saturated Fat, 3.5g Trans Fat), 160mg Sodium, 30mg Potassium, 1g Total Carbohydrate (1g Sugars), 1g Protein.
**Percent Daily Values are based on a 2,000 calories diet. Your daily values may be higher or lower depending on your calories needs:

Calories		2,000	2,500
Total Fat	Less than	65g	80g
Sat Fat	Less than	20g	25g
Cholesterol	Less than	300mg	300mg
Sodium	Less than	2400mg	2400mg
Potassium		3500mg	3500mg
Total Carbohydrate		300g	375g
Dietary Fiber		25g	30g

Calories per gram:
Fat 9   *   Carbohydrate 4   *   Protein 4

INTERPRETING THIS LABEL

At a glance the bottom third of it is a description of the fact that the additives used in the preparation of the mix add a lot of calories and fat: the additives to prepare this mac and cheese according to the package directions are 4 tablespoons of butter and ¼ cup of 2% skim milk. Any deviation from that will of course change these numbers. I add less butter and less milk which makes the mac and cheese thicker and cheesier (on those RARE occasions when I make this atrocity!)

Also of great interest is the fact that the FDA has CHANGED the RDA amounts of Sodium and Potassium from the numbers I have been using over the past ten years. The old values I have been using indicated a 100% RDA for Sodium of 2900mg and they have lowered this to 2400mg which is actually a HUGE amount (500mg less than before.) And the new 100% RDA of Potassium is set at 3500mg up from 3200mg. Both do play similar roles as electrolytes and both are necessary in the nerve ending-to-muscle cell synapses. These numbers likely reflect the latest contributions from medical industry testing in which excess Sodium has a confirmed affect of raising blood pressure while increased Potassium lowers blood pressure. (Watch for the upcoming volume: "The Truth About… Lowering Blood Pressure Without Drugs.")

1) Serving Size 2.5oz (70g/about 1/3 box) – This is a critical part of the nutrition label that most people either ignore or fail to "Do the Math" with it to see how many calories of the product they are actually eating at a given sitting. It's an important consideration with this product because the directions are for preparing the ENTIRE BOX (by adding those 4 tablespoons of butter and ¼ cup of 2% SKIM MILK) and nobody I know is going to try to measure out 1/3 of the box.

2) Servings per Container about 3 – This is the key piece of information in the header of the label. If you are consuming the whole container in one sitting then this tells you the MULTIPLIER for ALL of the values listed below and we will be multiplying everything by 3.

3) Amount per Serving… Mix… Prepared – These column headers point out the amount of the item and distinguish between the raw contents of the package and the cooked contents FOLLOWING the DIRECTIONS and the AMOUNTS of the suggested ingredients to be added. Any deviation will change the values in the "Prepared" column possibly SIGNFICANTLY.

I should point out that this particular food label has the added complication of the fact that it is a MIX and you must add other ingredients and that our choices of the amounts and kinds of ingredients that you add will change the numbers of the final product that you eat. Most products that are "Ready-to-Eat" do not have this second column of values and are thus much easier to read. I chose this label to give you a good example of one of the more complicated nutrition labels.

4) Calories… 250… 400 – Remember that they are using ONE serving for these numbers but we will use the entire box so we have to multiply EVERYTHIING by 3: the WHOLE BOX contains 750 calories and prepared the way they suggest in the directions will yield a pot of mac and cheese with a total content of 1200 calories.

5) Calories from Fat… 10… 150 – Clearly the MIX doesn't bring very much fat, but the butter and milk, whatever kinds and amounts you use, certainly will bring most of the fat in the final mac and cheese that you sit down to eat: 30 calories in the WHOLE BOX MIX, and an estimated 450 calories from fat in the final cooked whole box. Since you can't eat it raw, you have no choice but to add butter and milk which will bring up the amount of fat in the final cooked product.

5) % Daily Value** – Now they will tell you what percent of each item this food will bring with the understanding that your daily total should be near 100% without going over for harmful items like Saturated Fat and Cholesterol and you can go over for good items like safe vitamins. The double asterisk leads to a point underneath the lists which I will discuss when we get to it.

6) Total Fat 1g*… 2%… 26% – This row points out again that the MIX itself is not bringing very much fat but the butter and the milk certainly will. The asterisk leads to an explanation of this further down in the food label which I will elaborate on when we get to it. Don't forget to multiply that 26% by 3 = 78%. This one item will give you over ¾ of our daily allowance of fat. So you better not eat any other food with fat in it for the rest of the day!

7) Saturated Fat… 0%… 15% – This product contains no saturated fat but because we must use butter and milk it forces us to introduce about 15% of our daily allowance PER SERVING so TIMES 3 = 45%, nearly half of what we should eat daily in this one item.

8) Trans Fat 0g – This has no RDA because it is ARTIFICIAL and TOXIC. Be glad this product has none in it but your ARTIFICIAL BUTTER could be LOADED WITH IT. And dumping 4 table spoons into the pot could be terrible for your HEART HEALTH.

9) Cholesterol 0g… 0%… 0% – While the product brings none, this assumes that BOTH the butter you have chosen and the milk that you have chosen do not contain any cholesterol which is not necessarily true. BOTH of my choices DO have cholesterol in them.

10) Sodium 580mg… 24%… 31% – This is exactly why the medical industry first went on its anti-salt crusade, because food manufacturers are DUMPING MASSIVE AMOUNTS of POOR QUALITY SALT into EVERYTHING they make. This product is OVERLOADED with it and the WHOLE BOX contains 72% of your daily requirement of Sodium by itself. Because of this you cannot use IODIZED SALT or SEA SALT to help get our IODINE because you have already loaded up on Sodium in this product. This is the #1 REASON NOT to eat packaged products like this unless they are LOW SODIUM VERSIONS (very difficult to find in cooking mix products, by the way.)

11) Potassium 160g… 5%… 5% – It would have been far better for us if the manufacturer had bothered to add a boat load of Potassium salt rather than plain GARBAGE Sodium salt, but they didn't obviously. Nevertheless we do need a lot of Potassium so this one is a welcome sight even though the WHOLE box will only provide you with 15% of the RDA for this important mineral.

12) Total Carbohydrate 52g… 17%… 18% – There is a trick to this one. They have already discussed the fats separately and two lines down they reveal the amount of sugars (a carbohydrate) as 2g (2 grams) while this line says 52g. So what are these other 50 grams of carbohydrates in this food? STARCH which is the very definition of TRASH CALORIES that no one should be eating. They come from the wheat flour in the macaroni pasta in the package. We DO need calories, but not a boat load of TRASH CALORIES. The best form of calories you can get from your foods is natural sugars (but not that processed white crystal GARBAGE) and UNREFINED POLYUNSATURATED fats (found in seeds and nuts which are high in essential nutrients and WORTH the calories in these forms) and SOME PROTEIN, but NO SATURATED FAT and NO STARCH. Multiply by 3 so this box is providing 51% of your DAILY CALORIC intake as STARCH.

13) Dietary Fiber 2g… 8%… 8% – Fiber comes from plants and it is the wheat flour in the pasta that is bringing all of this fiber. Fiber is good for you but the rest of the contents of this product make this food so bad that it isn't worth the few things that are actually good in it.

14) Protein 8g – This one needs a little explanation as well. First, there is no set RDA for protein in general although the FDA does recommend a minimum of 110g of Complete Protein (contains all nine essential amino acids) and this protein is coming from the pasta made from wheat and eggs. So we do not know how much of this is Complete Protein and the manufacturer is not obligated to tell us either. Expect most of it to be wheat protein (i.e. GLUTEN.) We also have to multiply by 3 so the box provides 24g of poor quality protein and down at the bottom they mention that there is roughly 4 calories in each gram of protein so this totals 96 calories from protein. We do not add it to the totals above, it is already included in those numbers.

15) Vitamin A… 0%… 15% – Finally, we have come to the part of the nutrition label that actually deals with NUTRITION! And the first item, Vitamin A, is ONLY coming from the milk that we provide and the entire box contains ZERO.

16) Vitamin C… 0%... 0% – Well, not even the milk helps with this critical nutrient. A TOTAL ZERO as far as Vitamin C goes. I can already think of a dozen side dishes for dinner that are FAR healthier than this nonsense: 4 oz of cabbage will provide less than 50 calories AND 100% RDA of Vitamin C.

17) Calcium… 2%... 4% – While there is a little calcium in both the package and the milk you provide, it will not be nearly enough to meet your daily requirements even though this product does bring a boat load of TRASH CALORIES which will prevent you from adding GOOD natural whole foods that WILL bring you the calcium you need.

18) Iron… 10%... 10% – The whole package will bring you 30% of your RDA for this critical nutrient, but where will you get the rest especially when this package cost you a lot of TRASH calories?

19) Folic Acid… 35%... 35% – Folates are very difficult to find and wheat, especially whole grain products and wheat germ are some of the best sources. Even though the whole box does provide you with just over 100% of this important vitamin, the cost in TRASH calories and Sodium doesn't justify it at all.

20) *Amount in mix. Prepared contributes an additional 150… – This line explains that all of the calories and fats are coming from the milk you provide and NOT their product.

21) **Percent Daily Values are based on a 2,000 calories diet… – This line and the rest of the label explains that the percentages are based on a diet of 2,000 calories per day and then they lay that out and compare it to a diet of 2,500 calories per day showing you the TOTALS of each type of nutrient that are recommended. It is all good information but let's be clear: we all know we need to stay away from: Sodium, Saturated Fat, and Cholesterol. The "recommended" amounts of these in the 2,000 calorie per day diet that they line up is CONFUSING. It doesn't mean that you should eat those amounts it means these should be maximums and that you should try to stay BELOW those amounts as much as possible.

WHAT HAVE YOU LEARNED?

The nutrient label is FAR from a nutrient label any more. There was no discussion of Zinc or Thiamine, Riboflavin, Niacin, etc. all of which are just as important as Vitamin A, C, Calcium and Iron. They are far more worried about warning you about the amounts of Saturated Fats and Cholesterol in your foods and still can't be clear about the fact that you simply need to avoid these at all costs and be done with it. I showed you how to calculate the ACTUAL amount of calories in a container (cals per serving TIMES the number of servings) and how to calculate the STARCH content and the fact that you should AVOID starch as much as possible: it is the PLANT EQUIVALENT of SATURATED FAT; you DON'T NEED IT. In the next chapter I will show you how to do a LOT more math on this nutrition label and it is an EYE opener.

So far you have been armed with many highly available superfoods as well as a cross reference so that you can quickly find a given nutrient and then those superfoods that can provide it. You have also been given some of the best online resources (last chapter) for finding foods as well as their detailed nutrition fact sheets and how to read those as well. The final piece of the puzzle is how to determine nutrient density in terms of calories per percent of a given nutrient (this tells you how many calories of the given food you need to eat in order to meet your RDA target amount per day) and the cost per percent of the nutrient (this tells you if you can afford it.) And both of these numbers are quite important indeed.

It is one thing to know that a given superfood will provide you with plenty of the nutrient but if you have to consume 2000 calories of it during the day to get 100% RDA of the nutrient, then it is not worth it because 2000 calories is all you should eat during the day and you might get bored eating this one item and nothing else, not to mention you will miss out on all of the other essential nutrients that it lacks. And if a food does provide what you want in a reasonable amount of calories but would also end up costing you even $10 a day, that could be a problem for a lot of people including myself – I can't afford to spend $300/month trying to get even several nutrients in one food and quite often I have run into this problem and had to back out of a specific food because it turned out to be too expensive to use as my primary source of a given nutrient.

I'll demonstrate both nutrient densities (that's cals/percent of nutrient X, and cost/percent of nutrient X) for several different foods for a couple of different nutrients so you can see how easy the math is. Don't get discouraged if it makes your head spin at first: you will get used to it with a little practice.

NUTRIENT DENSITY – CALORIES PER PERCENT

This calculation is very important because we want to make sure that the food we are considering will provide the desired nutrient without bringing so many calories that it really isn't worth it. That, in fact, is the entire purpose of the superfoods and the fact that they bring such high quantities of their nutrients means that they are the densest sources of them and that is exactly what makes them superfoods. In other words, practically all foods have traces of just about every essential nutrient, but if one ounce of the food brings 1% of a given nutrient, then you would be forced to eat 100 oz (over SIX POUNDS) of it to get the 100% RDA amount and that by itself is not only impractical, it is impossible. However, some superfoods that do bring a lot of the nutrient are also quite high in calories like the seeds and nuts. Even though you can eat a reasonable portion size in order to get the amount of the nutrient you seek, it may also add up to so many calories that you might decide to pass on it and that is why you must learn how to do this calculation.

STEP 1: Choose a nutrient. For this example I will choose Zinc which is very difficult to get from natural whole foods at 100% RDA amounts on a daily basis.

STEP 2: Find the foods that are richest in the nutrient. For Zinc we have Lamb at 15%RDA per ounce, Swiss Cheese 8% per ounce, Sunflower seed kernels 10% per ounce, and Pumpkin seeds 19% per ounce. (I am skipping the oysters which are hands down the very best source of Zinc at 170% RDA per oz. just for this exercise and because I don't want to eat them daily.)

STEP 3: Record how many calories per ounce each food has. For Lamb it is 68cal/ounce, Swiss cheese is 106cal/oz, sunflower seed kernels are 163cal/oz, and pumpkin seeds are 125cal/oz.

Without doing any math it is already clear that lamb has a decent percentage of Zinc per ounce and the lowest calories per ounce and is likely the highest density natural whole food source of Zinc, but sometimes the numbers can be deceiving which is why it is important to "do the math" anyway just to be sure.

STEP 4: Divide the number of calories in one ounce by the percentage of the nutrient in one ounce. So for lamb this is 68 / 15 = 4.533 and this is lamb's nutrient density of Zinc in terms of calories per percent of Zinc. In order to get 100% RDA amount of Zinc you would have to eat 4.533 x 100 = 453.3 calories of lamb meat which is quite reasonable in terms of caloric intake. Just remember that it is still going to take about 7.5 ounces of it per day which is quite a lot of meat. I have that kind of appetite, but a lot of people don't. Now let's do the Swiss cheese. 106 / 8 = 13.25 cal/% In order to get 100%: 13.25 x 100 = 1325cal. That is WAY TOO MUCH, it only leaves 775 calories of food for the rest of the day or well over half of the calories that you CAN eat during the day went into the cheese and it will take a little more than 12 ounces of it to reach the goal. Now let's try the sunflower seed kernels: 163 / 10 = 16.3 cal/%. So 16.3 x 100 = 1630 calories to get 100% of your Zinc making it WORSE than even the cheese. Finally, let's try the pumpkin seeds. 125 (cal/oz) divided by 19 (%) = 6.579 cal/%. So 6.579 x 100 = 657.9 calories need to be consumed in order to get 100% RDA of Zinc. This however only requires a little over five ounces of them.

CONCLUSION

Pumpkin seeds have the highest density by weight, that's what the nutrition tables give you, the highest percentage per ounce of the food: Pumpkin seeds 19%, Lamb meat 15%, Sunflower seeds 10%, and Swiss cheese 8%. So we already knew that we would have to eat the least amount by weight of the Pumpkin seeds to meet the 100% RDA amount. However, the Lamb meat has the lowest density in terms of how many

CALORIES of it we have to consume in order to meet the 100% RDA amount of Zinc. Therefore Lamb meat has the highest nutrient density of Zinc in terms of calories per percent of all foods for which we did the math here. One last interesting observation: pumpkin seeds are actually quite light, five ounces would be slightly more than two liquid measuring cups of them. That is a lot of VOLUME and eating all of that food will bring a lot of fiber and fill your stomach up before most people could finish them off. The lamb meat on the other hand is quite dense in terms of weight per unit volume and 7.5 ounces is a rather small steak. Finally, oysters blow all of the other sources of Zinc out of the water; they are BY FAR the densest source of Zinc possible; 1oz brings 170%DV.

NUTRIENT DENSITY – COST PER PERCENT

This calculation is just as important. It makes no sense to settle on a food that will provide a nutrient in a reasonable portion size that is also low in calories only to realize that it costs so much that it simply isn't practical. One of the criteria I used to choose the superfoods was that they had to be fairly common and therefore more than likely affordable as well. I never bothered to check the nutrition fact sheets of caviar or lobster because I certainly can't afford to eat either one of those on a daily basis. If you can, then you can check their nutrient fact sheets and apply these formulas and it might turn out that these foods will fill your nutrient requirements and fit your budget and that would be splendid. For the rest of us working stiffs, we will need to do a little more math. For this example I am going to try to fulfill my daily requirement of calcium with natural whole foods.

STEP 1: I can't find solid block parmesan cheese at my local grocery stores, but they do have grated parmesan for sprinkling on pasta so I will test this product. $2.99 buys an 8 ounce shaker of it at my local store. But most stores including this one show you the cost per ounce right on the shelf price label and that makes this project a LOT easier. If you don't know the price per ounce I will include the calculation in Step 2, if you do know the price per ounce you can skip to Step 3. I am going to compare the Parmesan to a block of Swiss cheese and boxed whole milk as well. The Swiss is available as an 8 ounce block for $3.29 and the boxed whole milk is at the dollar store for $1 for 32 ounces.

STEP 2: To get the price per ounce divide the total price of the food by the number of ounces it contains. So the Parmesan is $2.99, but I will round it to $3, so ($) 3 / 8 (oz.) = 0.375 dollars / oz. Multiply by 100 = 37.5 cents/oz. The Swiss is 3.29 / 8 = 0.41125 dollars/oz or 41.12 cents/oz. And the milk is ($) 1 / 32 = 0.03125 dollars per ounce x 100 = 3.125 cents per oz.

STEP 3: The packaging of the Parmesan says that a serving contains 6% of my daily requirement of Calcium based on a 2000 calorie per day diet. We know they mean 6% of 1000mg and the serving size is 5g. We know that Parmesan and Romano are about the same and you can use the numbers I have provided in the section on the superfoods, but let's use what the packaging says so we are completely accurate about THIS particular product. The exact conversion of grams to ounces is about 28.35 grams per ounce. But we can keep this simple and just call it 28. So 28 divided by 5 (the given serving size) = 5.6 and we now multiply this by the 6%: 5.6 x 6 = 33.6% calcium per ounce which is almost the same as the value in the superfoods section of this book. Now let's do this calculation for the Swiss cheese. This product made life a lot easier since the serving size on the package says 1 ounce and the amount of calcium per serving is listed as 22% which is also right in line with the value provided in the superfoods chapter. The milk calls the serving size 8 ounces and amount of calcium provided is 30%. So how much calcium per ounce? 30 divided by 8 = 3.75. So the Parmesan provides 33.6%/oz, the Swiss is 22%/oz and the milk is 3.75%/oz.

STEP 4: We need the cost of the calcium per percentage point. Now we divide the cost per ounce by the percent per ounce and this will yield the cost per percent: Parmesan: 37.5 (cents/oz) / 33.6 (%/oz) = 1.116 cents / % calcium. Swiss cheese: 41.12 / 22 = 1.869 cents / % calcium. Boxed Whole Milk: 3.125 / 3.75 = 0.833 cents per % calcium.

STEP 5: Now how much does it cost per day to get 100% RDA of calcium from each product? Parmesan: 1.116 cents / % just change the value to dollars and drop the "/%" so it costs $1.12 (I set this up like this on purpose!) Swiss: $1.87 and the milk: $0.83.

CONCLUSION

So even though the milk has the lowest percentage of calcium per ounce, it is also so much cheaper that it does work out to be the cheapest product to provide 100% RDA of calcium: just 83 cents per day. However, at 3.75% / oz. it is also going to take 100 / 3.75 = 26.66 ounces to do it. If you are fine with drinking that much milk each day, then go for it, but keep in mind that the milk also says that it has 150 calories per 8 oz serving. 26.66 / 8 = 3.33. This number times those 150 calories is 500 calories per day in milk alone to get 100% RDA off calcium. Most of those calories are due to the fat so skim milk would be preferable even if it has lower amounts of calcium in it. The Parmesan is 20 cal per 5g serving so 28 (g/oz) divided by 5g = 5.6 x 20 cal = 112 cal per oz. 3 oz will make 100% RDA so 112 x 3 = 336 calories to get 100% RDA calcium from Parmesan cheese. The Swiss package says 110 cal per 1 oz. serving and it will take 100(%) divided by 22(%/oz) = 4.5 oz to get 100% calcium. 4.5 x 112 = 504. Processed low fat cheeses are of greatly inferior quality as is skim milk by the way. Since all of these products are relatively unprocessed (they are not low fat versions) it turns out that the Parmesan is the best in terms of calories required to consume 100% RDA of calcium, while the milk is the cheapest. The Swiss is the worst in terms of calories required to reach 100% RDA calcium and it is the most expensive as well.

So how do I get my calcium? Calcium is a tough one to get in 100% RDA amounts on a daily basis. I drink two 8 oz. café con leche drinks each day (that's 16 oz of the whole milk which provides 60% of the RDA of calcium) and I follow that up at some point with 2 ounces of dollar store bought Pepperjack cheese which provides 20% RDA of calcium per ounce to get my other 40%. Total cost for the day? 50 cents for the milk and 33 cents for the cheese ($1 for a six ounce slab which I cut into thirds of 2 ounces each.) Sometimes you have to shop around and you also have to make decisions about what foods you are willing to consume in the amounts necessary to make the RDA amount. I already drink far too much coffee anyway, so by converting two servings during the day into café con leche which brings the much needed whole milk I have turned them into HEALTHY choices, they at least bring that calcium along with them. The rest can be taken care of with a relatively small amount of any cheese I just chose the cheapest one I could find at the dollar store. But READ THE LABELS! I bought some individually wrapped "Swiss cheese" at the dollar store and found out it had no calcium in it because it wasn't cheese at all – just fake slices made out of hydrogenated vegetable oil!

A RECAP OF THE CONVERSIONS

Cal per percent of nutrient X = cal/oz divided by percentage/oz
EXAMPLE: A food has 14% of nutrient X and is 90 calories per ounce: 90(cal/oz) divided by 14(% of X) = 6.428 cal / %
IF the percentage or serving size is given in grams: the calculation still works because the serving size has been removed from the number which expresses calories per percentage RDA of the nutrient. 10% of X in 14g serving of 16 cals: 16/10 = 1.6cal / %.
Cost per percent of nutrient X: cost per ounce (in cents) divided by the percent per ounce.
EXAMPLE: A food costs 25 cents/oz and provides 10% RDA of the nutrient per ounce therefore: 25 / 10 = 2.5 cents/% which equals $2.50 for 100% RDA of the nutrient.
Converting grams/serving to 1oz: 28 divided by serving size in grams:
EXAMPLE: A food provides 23% of nutrient X in a serving size of 35g and costs 40 cents per oz.:
Step 1) Convert to ounces by dividing 28 by the given serving size in grams: 28 / 35 = 0.8.
Step 2) Then multiply by the percentage of the nutrient provided by the value obtained in step 1: 0.8 x 23(%) = 18.4%/oz.
Step 3) Divide cents per ounce by the percentage of nutrient provided per ounce: 40 / 18.4 = 2.174 cents / % or $2.17 for 100% RDA of nutrient X per day.

MORE EXAMPLES
EXAMPLE 1:

Calculate the nutrient density in cals/oz and cost/% of Zinc provided by oysters given they cost $2 for an 8 oz can and provide 170% Zinc per ounce and are 19.3 calories per oz.

Oysters (canned): 170% Zinc / oz, 19.3 cal / oz and $2 for 8 oz

Nutrient Density in cal/% Zinc: cal / oz divided by %Zinc / oz.

    19.3 / 170 = 0.1135. Multiply by 100:

    11.35 calories brings 100% RDA of Zinc.

Nutrient Cost in cents / % Zinc: Find the cost of 1 oz: Divide the cost of the product by the weight in oz: $2 / 8 oz = $0.25 or 25 cents / oz. Now cost / oz divided by % Zinc / oz gives the cost per percent: 25 (cents/oz) / 170 (% Zinc/oz.) = 0.147 cents / %. Drop the "/ %" and you get:

    $0.147 or $0.15 (15 cents) to get 100% RDA of Zinc.

EXAMPLE 2:

Which is the best source of Vitamin C; Cabbage or Grapefruit?
Step 1) Amounts per oz. Cabbage: 24%/oz, Grapefruit: 15%/oz (from the tables in the Superfoods chapter.)
Step 2) At my local grocery store cabbage is normally 69 cents / pound and grapefruits are $3.99 for a five pound bag which usually holds eight medium sized grapefruits. ($) 4 / 8 fruits = 0.5 or 50 cents per grapefruit and each weighs: 5 (lb) / 8 = 0.625 lb. Multiply by 16 (oz/lb) = 10 ounces. 1 small cabbage weighs about 2.25 lb x 0.69 = $1.55 for a small cabbage. ¼ of that cabbage head weighs about 8 oz.
Step 3) One grapefruit costs 50 cents and weighs 10 ounces. It brings 10 (oz) x 15 (% Vitamin C) = 150% Vitamin C. ¼ small head of cabbage weighs 8 oz, costs about 40 cents and brings 8 (oz) x 24 (% Vitamin C) = 192% Vitamin C.
CONCLUSION:

    The cabbage is CHEAPER, 40 cents per convenient serving versus 50 cents per grapefruit and brings MORE Vitamin C in a slightly smaller serving. 8 oz x 6.7 cal/oz = 53.6 calories of cabbage to get 192% Vitamin C and 10 oz x 11.8 cal/oz = 118 calories of grapefruit to get 150% Vitamin C. The cabbage is denser in terms of cal/percent of Vitamin C as well. Therefore, cabbage is cheaper and has a higher nutrient density of Vitamin C than grapefruit. And no one ever believes me until I do the math!

A LITTLE MORE PRACTICE

EXAMPLE: Calculate the nutrient density in calories and cost of the top two available sources of Iron: Canned Clams and Baker's Chocolate.

Clams: 41.4 cal/oz, 43% Iron per oz. and 6.5 oz. can costs $1.69

Nutrient Density in cal/% Iron: cal / oz divided by %Iron / oz.

    41.4 / 43 = 0.96. About 1 cal per percent of Iron so:

    100 calories brings 100% RDA of Iron.

67

Nutrient Cost in cents / % Iron: Find the cost of 1 oz: Divide the
cost of the product by the weight in oz: $1.69 / 6.5 oz = $0.26
or 26 cents / oz. Now cost / oz divided by % Iron / oz gives the
cost per percent: 26 (cents/oz) / 43 (% Iron/oz.) = 0.604 cents
/ %. Drop the "/ %" and you get:
$0.60 to get 100% RDA of Iron.

Baker's Chocolate: 140 cal / oz, 27% Iron / oz, and $2 for 4 oz.

Nutrient Density in cal/% Iron: cal / oz divided by %Iron / oz.
140 / 27 = 5.185 Multiply this by 100:
518.5 calories brings 100% RDA of Iron.

Nutrient Cost in cents / % Iron: Find the cost of 1 oz: Divide the
cost of the product by the weight in oz: $2 / 4 oz = $0.50 or 50
cents / oz. Now cost / oz divided by % Iron / oz gives the cost
per percent: 50 (cents/oz) / 27 (% Iron/oz.) = 1.851 cents / %.
Drop the "/ %" and you get:
$1.85 to get 100% RDA of Iron.

Clams are over FIVE TIMES DENSER in Iron in terms of calories
required in order to get 100% RDA of Iron (it takes over five times
the calories to get 100% RDA amount from the chocolate) and
they are also ONE THIRD the cost (60 cents versus $1.85)
EXAMPLE 2: Calculate the actual nutrient density in cal/oz and
cost/% of Zinc in Oysters

USING ORAC SCORES

Quite often I compare foods based on their ORAC scores by
comparing them to raw carrots. I always assume that an average
carrot weighs about 4 oz. So let's compare and 8 oz. cup of freshly
squeezed Pomegranate Juice to the carrots:
STEP 1) EQUALIZE THE AMOUNTS FIRST: Since the cup of
Pomegranate Juice is 8 oz (all liquids can be considered 8 oz per
cup) it is DOUBLE the weight; So multiply the Pomegranate ORAC
Score by 2: 55520 x 2 = 111040
STEP 2: Divide the substance being compared, by the ORAC
Score of the raw carrots (697): 111040 / 697 = 159.311. The cup
of juice has the antioxidant power of 160 carrots or about 40
pounds of them. Bear in mind that the juice is NOT the same
potency as eating the whole fruit especially with Pomegranates,
but they are still much higher in antioxidant potential than any
other fruit juice except Açai.
EXAMPLE 2: Compare Black Pepper to Carrots.
STEP 1) Half a teaspoon is about 1.2g and one carrot is 28 g/oz X
4oz = 112g. divide 1.2 by 112 = 0.0107. This is the number to
multiply to the black pepper ORAC Score: 34053 x 0.0107 = 364.3
STEP 2) Divide this by the ORAC Score of the raw carrots (697) =
364.3 / 697 = 0.5226
CONCLUSION) Just ½ teaspoon of black pepper has the
antioxidant power of about half a raw carrot; not bad for such a tiny
amount! And ½ teaspoon of a spice with an ORAC score twice as
high (around 70,000) would be equivalent to one whole carrot.

You know the old saying, "Give a man a fish…" These books are basically those "fish" that I am giving to you, now I am going to show you HOW to fish for yourself: the best sources of information and how to use that information; how to apply it to your daily healthy dietary regimen.

Before we begin I should mention that I have not contacted these websites and I don't think I own stock in any of them either. (I have an old penny stock account somewhere, I can't even remember where, much less the password or what I own.) The point is that all of these are included because they are reliable and useful sources of information that I have used in writing these books and I will show you how to use their information for yourself.

As long as you are sticking to a natural whole foods diet (buying almost everything from the fresh produce section and the fresh meat/dairy sections of your local grocery store then you are definitely on the right track, but many essential nutrients are rather hard to find in sufficient quantities in most foods. So even if you are eating right, you might still fall short on many essential nutrients like Vitamin B2 – Riboflavin, as well as B9 – Folic acid and Choline not to mention Chromium and Magnesium to name a handful of essential vitamins and minerals that are hard to get even from a natural whole foods diet in at least 100% RDA amounts on a daily basis. And don't forget that the FDA's RDA values are conservative one-size fits all ESTIMATES and we all know that women need more iron than men, and hard working men need more of almost everything than seven year old kids.

THE FDA and the NIH

Both of these governmental agencies (the Food and Drug Administration and the National Institutes of Health) have very good and informative websites. Like all governmental agencies their websites can be difficult to navigate and the material is often either too simplified or too complicated to be of much value, but I still recommend that you visit them and take a look around.

The U.S. Food and Drug Administration: www.fda.gov

The National Institutes for Health: www.nih.gov

"DR. AXE"

This is an extensive website which I have used as a primary base source of most of the information on the essential nutrients that includes excellent explanations of what each nutrient is, the health benefits of each one, the nasty results of chronic deficiency for each one, and a list of foods that contain them. The website covers a lot of ground too, not just the "ABC's" (the vitamins and minerals) but also many other health food items and supplements like lycopene, Milk Thistle, and fad products like Creatine, etc. This website comes highly recommended.

Dr. Axe: www.draxe.com

"MYFOODDATA"

This is another superb website although they don't get too deep into the nature of each nutrient and it is far from complete like "Dr. Axe" but they do have excellent lists of the top foods that contain each essential nutrient that they do cover and it is a good source of that specific information and I highly recommend that you check it out too.

WEBSITE ADDRESS: www.myfooddata.com

THE GEORGE MATELJAN FOUNDATION

This is another excellent reference website that covers many minerals that most other websites do not. They include a lot of good information on the function of most of the nutrients in the human body as well, some of which I could only find at this website.

WEBSITE ADDRESS: www.whfoods.com

WIKIPEDIA

Often maligned because "anybody" can start an entry or edit an existing entry, Wikipedia is by far the largest repository of general information on every conceivable subject on planet Earth. It is an enormous encyclopedia and while some entries on the subject of nutrients are rather limited and also include a lot of talk about the molecular structures, and chemistry like methods of synthesis and so on, it is still one of the best online resources that covers everything and each page does include the references which you can pursue as well. Whenever they ask for a few dollars, please give, so we can keep this vast repository of information free and unencumbered by advertising.

WEBSITE ADDRESS: www.wikipedia.org

"SUPERFOODLY"

This website lists the ORAC – Oxygen Radical Absorption Capacity – scores for many different foods, mostly natural whole foods. While the ORAC score was invented to try to measure the antioxidant potential of foods compared to each other side-by-side (the ORAC score is based on 100 grams of each food) it is not absolute. All antioxidants are not the same. Some are found in the nucleus of cells like Vitamin E which plays a role in the maintenance and replication of DNA, while others are involved in countless cellular chemical processes like Vitamin C while others freely wander in the bloodstream neutralizing free radicals there as well. And each antioxidant has a different affinity (the precise free radicals that it prefers to neutralize) and potency (some can neutralize lots of free radicals while others get "spent" after neutralizing just a few or even just one free radical, but that does not mean that they are less effective if that job was performed in the nucleus of the cell directly in the defense of the DNA and therefore prevented corruption of that DNA which could lead directly to cancer. And this does not diminish the importance of the ORAC scores either. The thing to remember is not to use the information to replace one food item with another, but to add powerful antioxidant-rich foods to your regular eating regimen. For example, cloves have one of the highest scores of all foods, about 290,000 while carrots have an ORAC score of about 700. But you can't replace a medium sized carrot with a gram of cloves because the carrots bring beta-carotene which for many people is the only way they are going to get their daily requirement of Vitamin A which the body can easily generate from the beta-carotene. I highly recommend this website as a way to "shop for" new antioxidant-rich foods to add to your regular natural whole foods diet just like I do.

WEBSITE ADDRESS: www.superfoodly.com

NUTRITION DATA at SELF.COM

I am not sure if I could even write this volume of the series without this website. They have one of the largest repositories of detailed chemical nutrient analyses of every possible food, both packaged as well as natural whole foods, imaginable. You can literally search for ANY FOOD you can think of and they will have its complete nutrition label including every vitamin, mineral, and many other nutrients as well as "undesirable" constituents listed in that label. I have this one bookmarked so I can quickly check the nutritional value of any food at any time.

WEBSITE ADDRESS: http://nutritiondata.self.com

"WEB MD"

Aside from having an extensive collection of articles on the nutrients, WebMD also includes many excellent articles on prevention and treatment for many ailments and afflictions as well. I could not remember where I had heard the TRUTH ABOUT turkey causing drowsiness after Thanksgiving dinner – that this effect is caused by the high levels of LACTIC ACID in Turkey meat and the extreme overindulgence of it at the Thanksgiving table and that it is NOT caused by Tryptophan. In a general google search, WebMD was near the top of the list with an article that confirmed that Tryptophan – an ESSENTIAL AMINO ACID found in ALL PROTEINS in ALL CELLS in YOUR BODY and with HIGHER CONCENTRATIONS in CHICKEN than Turkey – is NOT the cause of drowsiness EVER: OVEREATING Complete Protein (animal source protein) is the cause they lay out and I still can't find where I read that it was the lactic acid! But the point is that WebMD is a great source of health related information and I definitely have it bookmarked on all of my computers.

WEBSITE ADDRESS: www.webmd.com

THANK YOU AND GOD BLESS AND GOOD LUCK AND ABOVE ALL ELSE; TAKE CARE OF YOURSELF (BECAUSE NO ONE ELSE IS GOING TO DO IT!)

REFERENCES

[1] Omega-3 fatty acids: https://draxe.com/omega-3-benefits-plus-top-10-omega-3-foods-list/ Retrieved on 8/23/18

[2] Atlantic Mackerel: https://nutritiondata.self.com/facts/finfish-and-shellfish-products/4072/2 Retrieved on 9/12/18

[3] Tuna: https://nutritiondata.self.com/facts/finfish-and-shellfish-products/4206/2 Retrieved on 9/12/18

[4] Vitamin B12: https://draxe.com/vitamin-b12/benefits/ Retrieved on 7/24/18 * https://en.wikipedia.org/wiki/Cobalamin Retrieved on 7/24/18

[5] Selenium: * https://draxe.com/selenium-foods/ Retrieved on 8/23/18 * https://www.myfooddata.com/articles/foods-high-in-selenium.php Retrieved on /8/23/18 * http://www.whfoods.com/genpage.php?tname=nutrient&dbid=95 Retrieved on 8/23/18

[6] Salmon: https://nutritiondata.self.com/facts/ethnic-foods/10460/2 Retrieved on 9/12/18

[7] Vitamin B7 – Biotin: https://draxe.com/biotin-benefits/ Retrieved on 7/24/18 * https://en.wikipedia.org/wiki/Biotin Retrieved on 7/24/18

[8] Astaxanthin: Rachael Link, MS, RD, https://draxe.com/astaxanthin-benefits/ Retrieved on 8/20/18

[9] Sardines: https://nutritiondata.self.com/facts/finfish-and-shellfish-products/4114/2 Retrieved on 9/12/18

[10] Oysters: https://nutritiondata.self.com/facts/finfish-and-shellfish-products/4192/2 Retrieved on 9/12/18

[11] Zinc: https://draxe.com/foods-high-in-zinc/ Retrieved on 8/23/18 * https://www.myfooddata.com/articles/high-zinc-foods.php Retrieved on 8/23/18 * http://www.whfoods.com/genpage.php?tname=nutrient&dbid=115 Retrieved on 8/23/18

[12] Clams: https://nutritiondata.self.com/facts/finfish-and-shellfish-products/4183/2 Retrieved on 9/12/18

[13] Iron: https://draxe.com/top-10-iron-rich-foods/ Retrieved on 7/30/18 * https://www.myfooddata.com/articles/food-sources-of-iron.php Retrieved on 7/30/18 * http://www.whfoods.com/genpage.php?tname=nutrient&dbid=70 Retrieved on 7/30/18

[14] Vitamin B2 – Riboflavin: https://draxe.com/vitamin-b2/ Retrieved on 7/23/18 * http://www.whfoods.com/genpage.php?tname=nutrient&dbid=93 Retrieved on 7/23/18 * https://www.myfooddata.com/articles/foods-high-in-riboflavin-vitamin-B2.php Retrieved on 7/23/18 * https://ods.od.nih.gov/factsheets/Riboflavin-HealthProfessional/ Retrieved on 7/23/18

[15] Lamb: https://nutritiondata.self.com/facts/lamb-veal-and-game-products/4474/2 Retrieved on 9/12/18

[16] Vitamin A: https://draxe.com/top-10-vitamin-foods/ Retrieved on 7/23/18 * https://www.myfooddata.com/articles/food-sources-of-vitamin-A.php Retrieved on 7/23/18 * http://www.whfoods.com/genpage.php?tname=nutrient&dbid=106 Retrieved on 7/23/18

[17] Choline: https://draxe.com/what-is-choline/ Retrieved on 7/24/18 * http://www.whfoods.com/genpage.php?tname=nutrient&dbid=50 Retrieved on 7/24/18

[18] Copper: https://draxe.com/foods-high-in-copper/ Retrieved on 8/23/18 * https://www.myfooddata.com/articles/high-copper-foods.php Retrieved on 8/23/18 * http://www.whfoods.com/genpage.php?tname=nutrient&dbid=53 Retrieved on 8/23/18

[19] Beef liver: https://nutritiondata.self.com/facts/beef-products/3468/2
    Retrieved on 9/12/18

[20] Turkey: https://nutritiondata.self.com/facts/poultry-products/931/2
    Retrieved on 9/12/18

[21] Calcium: https://draxe.com/foods-high-in-calcium/ Retrieved on
    7/30/18 * https://www.myfooddata.com/articles/foods-high-in-
    calcium.php Retrieved on 7/30/18 * http://www.whfoods.com/
    genpage.php?tname=nutrient&dbid=45 Retrieved on 7/30/18

[22] Parmesan (and Romano) cheese: https://nutritiondata.self.com/facts/
    dairy-and-egg-products/32/2 Retrieved on 9/12/18

[23] Phosphorus: https://draxe.com/foods-high-in-phosphorus/ Retrieved
    on 7/30/18 * https://www.myfooddata.com/articles/high-phosphorus-
    foods.php Retrieved on 7/30/18 * http://www.whfoods.com/
    genpage.php?tname=nutrient&dbid=127 Retrieved on 7/30/18

 [24] Swiss cheese: https://nutritiondata.self.com/facts/dairy-and-egg-
    products/39/2 Retrieved on 9/12/18

[25] Yogurt: https://nutritiondata.self.com/facts/dairy-and-egg-
    products/104/2 Retrieved on 9/12/18

[26] Vitamin D3 – Cholecalciferol: https://draxe.com/vitamin-d-deficiency-
    symptoms/ Retrieved on 7/28/18 * https://www.myfooddata.com/
    articles/high-vitamin-D-foods.php Retrieved on 7/28/18 *
    http://www.whfoods.com/genpage.php?tname=nutrient&dbid=110
    Retrieved on 7/28/18

[27] Cod Liver Oil: https://nutritiondata.self.com/facts/fats-and-oils/628/2
    Retrieved on 9/12/18

[28] Manganese: https://draxe.com/manganese/ Retrieved on 8/23/18
    * https://www.myfooddata.com/articles/foods-high-in-manganese.php
    Retrieved on 8/23/18

[29] Walnuts: https://nutritiondata.self.com/facts/nut-and-seed-
    products/3138/2 Retrieved on 9/12/18

[30] Fiber: https://draxe.com/high-fiber-foods/ Retrieved on 8/20/18

[31] Vitamin E – alpha-Tocopherol: https://draxe.com/vitamin-e-foods/
    Retrieved on 7/28/18 * https://www.myfooddata.com/articles/
    vitamin-e-foods.php Retrieved on 7/28/18 *
    http://www.whfoods.com/genpage.php?tname=nutrient&dbid=111
    Retrieved on 7/28/18

[32] Almonds: https://nutritiondata.self.com/facts/nut-and-seed-
    products/3087/2 Retrieved on 9/12/18

[33] Vitamin B1 – Thiamine: https://draxe.com/thiamine-foods/ Retrieved on
    7/23/18 * https://ods.od.nih.gov/factsheets/Thiamin-
    HealthProfessional/ Retrieved on 7/23/18

[34] Vitamin B3 – Niacin: https://draxe.com/niacin-side-effects/ Retrieved
    on 7/24/18 * https://www.myfooddata.com/articles/foods-high-in-
    niacin-vitamin-B3.php Retrieved on 7/24/18 *
    http://www.whfoods.com/genpage.php?tname=nutrient&dbid=83
    Retrieved on 7/24/18

[35] Vitamin B5 – Pantothenic acid: https://draxe.com/vitamin-b5/ Retrieved
    on 7/24/18 * http://www.whfoods.com/genpage.php?tname=
    nutrient&dbid=87 Retrieved on 7/24/18

[36] Vitamin B6 – Pyridoxine: https://draxe.com/top-10-vitamin-b6-foods/
    Retrieved on 7/24/18 * http://www.whfoods.com/genpage.php?
    tname=nutrient&dbid=108 Retrieved on 7/24/18

[37] Vitamin B9 – Folate: * https://draxe.com/top-10-vitamin-b9-folate-
    foods/ Retrieved on 7/24/18 * http://www.whfoods.com/

genpage.php?tname=nutrient&dbid=63 Retrieved on 7/24/18

[38] Magnesium: https://draxe.com/magnesium-deficient-top-10-magnesium-rich-foods-must-eating/ Retrieved on 7/30/18 * https://www.myfooddata.com/articles/foods-high-in-magnesium.php Retrieved on 7/30/18 * http://www.whfoods.com/genpage.php?tname=nutrient&dbid=75 Retrieved on 7/30/18

[39] Potassium: https://draxe.com/low-potassium/ Retrieved on 8/23/18 * https://www.myfooddata.com/articles/food-sources-of-potassium.php Retrieved on 8/23/18

[40] Sunflower seed kernels: https://nutritiondata.self.com/facts/nut-and-seed-products/3077/2 Retrieved on 9/12/18

[41] Pumpkin Seeds: https://nutritiondata.self.com/facts/nut-and-seed-products/3141/2 Retrieved on 9/12/18

[42] Brazil nuts: https://nutritiondata.self.com/facts/nut-and-seed-products/3091/2 Retrieved on 9/12/18

[43] Pistachio: https://nutritiondata.self.com/facts/nut-and-seed-products/3136/2 Retrieved on 9/12/18

[44] Vitamin K: https://draxe.com/vitamin-k-deficiency/ Retrieved on 7/28/18 * https://www.myfooddata.com/articles/food-sources-of-vitamin-k.php Retrieved on 7/28/18 * http://www.whfoods.com/genpage.php?tname=nutrient&dbid=112 Retrieved on 7/28/18

[45] Spinach: https://nutritiondata.self.com/facts/vegetables-and-vegetable-products/2626/2 Retrieved on 9/12/18

[46] Chlorophyll: https://draxe.com/chlorophyll-benefits/ Retrieved on 8/20/18 * https://en.wikipedia.org/wiki/Chlorophyll Retrieved on 8/20/18

[47] Zeaxanthin and Lutein: https://draxe.com/lutein/ Retrieved on 8/20/18 * https://en.wikipedia.org/wiki/Zeaxanthin Retrieved on 8/20/18

[48] Kale: https://nutritiondata.self.com/facts/vegetables-and-vegetable-products/2461/2 Retrieved on 9/12/18

[49] Vitamin C: https://draxe.com/vitamin-c-benefits/ Retrieved on 7/26-18 * https://www.myfooddata.com/articles/vitamin-c-foods.php Retrieved on 7/26-18 * http://www.whfoods.com/genpage.php?tname=nutrient&dbid=109 Retrieved on 7/26-18

[50] Lettuce: https://nutritiondata.self.com/facts/vegetables-and-vegetable-products/2476/2 Retrieved on 9/12/18

[51] Net Negative Calorie foods: https://nutritionfacts.org/18/06/07/foods-with-negative-calories/ Retrieved on 9/18/18 * https://food.ndtv.com/food-drinks/11-foods-that-burn-more-calories-than-they-contain-1679965 Retrieved on 9/18/18 * https://en.wikipedia.org/wiki/Negative-calorie_food Retrieved on 9/18/18

[52] Cabbage: https://nutritiondata.self.com/facts/vegetables-and-vegetable-products/2372/2 Retrieved on 9/12/18

[53] Carrots: https://nutritiondata.self.com/facts/vegetables-and-vegetable-products/2383/2 Retrieved on 9/12/18

[54] Apiole: https://en.wikipedia.org/wiki/Apiole Retrieved on 8/20/18

[55] Apigenin: https://en.wikipedia.org/wiki/Apigenin Retrieved on 8/20/18

[56] Celery: https://nutritiondata.self.com/facts/vegetables-and-vegetable-products/2396/2 Retrieved on 9/12/18

[57] Chromium: https://draxe.com/what-is-chromium/ Retrieved on 8/23/18 * http://www.whfoods.com/genpage.php?tname=nutrient&dbid=51 Retrieved on 8/23/18

[58] Broccoli: https://nutritiondata.self.com/facts/vegetables-and-vegetable-products/2356/2 Retrieved on 9/12/18

[59] Molybdenum: http://www.whfoods.com/genpage.php?tname=nutrient
&dbid=128 Retrieved on 8/29-18

[60] Chickpeas: https://nutritiondata.self.com/facts/legumes-and-legume-
products/4325/2 Retrieved on 9/12/18

[61] Lentils: https://nutritiondata.self.com/facts/legumes-and-legume-
products/4337/2 Retrieved on 9/12/18

[62] Green peas: https://nutritiondata.self.com/facts/vegetables-and-
vegetable-products/2888/2 Retrieved on 9/12/18

[63] Peanuts and peanut butter: https://nutritiondata.self.com/facts/
legumes-and-legume-products/4453/2 Retrieved on 9/12/18

[64] Saponins: https://en.wikipedia.org/wiki/Saponin Retrieved on 8/20/18

[65] Oats: https://nutritiondata.self.com/facts/breakfast-cereals/1597/2
Retrieved on 9/12/18

[66] Betaine: https://draxe.com/what-is-betaine/ Retrieved on 8/20/18 *
https://en.wikipedia.org/wiki/Betaine Retrieved on 8/20/18

[67] Alkylresorcinols: https://en.wikipedia.org/wiki/Alkylresorcinol Retrieved
on 8/20/18

[68] Wheat germ: https://nutritiondata.self.com/facts/cereal-grains-and-
pasta/5743/2 Retrieved on 9/12/18

[69] Banana: https://nutritiondata.self.com/facts/fruits-and-fruit-
juices/1846/2 Retrieved on 9/12/18

[70] Cucumbers: https://nutritiondata.self.com/facts/vegetables-and-
vegetable-products/2440/2 Retrieved on 9/12/18

[71] Grapefruit: https://nutritiondata.self.com/facts/fruits-and-fruit-
juices/1905/2 Retrieved on 9/12/18

[72] Resveratrol: https://draxe.com/all-about-resveratrol/ Retrieved on
8/20/18 * https://en.wikipedia.org/wiki/Resveratrol Retrieved on
8/20/18

[73] Myricetin: https://en.wikipedia.org/wiki/Myricetin Retrieved on 8/20/18

[74] Anthocyanidins: https://draxe.com/anthocyanin/ Retrieved on 8/20/18 *
https://en.wikipedia.org/wiki/Anthocyanidin Retrieved on 8/20/18

[75] Antioxidants: https://draxe.com/top-10-high-antioxidant-foods/
Retrieved on 8-20-18 * http://www.superfoodly.com (ORAC scores)
Retrieved on 8-29-18

[76] Grapes and grape juice: https://draxe.com/grapes-nutrition/ Retrieved
on 9/12/18

[77] Kiwi: https://nutritiondata.self.com/facts/fruits-and-fruit-juices/1934/2
Retrieved on 9/12/18

[78] Phenylethanoids: https://en.wikipedia.org/wiki/Phenylethanoid
Retrieved on 8/20/18

[79] Oleanolic acid: https://en.wikipedia.org/wiki/Oleanolic_acid Retrieved
on 8/20/18

[80] Olives: http://www.whfoods.com/genpage.php?tname=foodspice&
dbid=46 Retrieved on 9/18/18

[81] Lycopene: https://draxe.com/lycopene/ Retrieved on 8/20/18 *
https://en.wikipedia.org/wiki/Lycopene Retrieved on 8/20/18

[82] Tomatoes: https://nutritiondata.self.com/facts/vegetables-and-
vegetable-products/2682/2 Retrieved on 9/12/18

[83] ORAC Scores: http://www.superfoodly.com Retrieved on 8-29-18

[84] Catechins: https://en.wikipedia.org/wiki/Catechin Retrieved on 8/20/18

[85] Cinnamon: https://www.healthline.com/nutrition/10-proven-benefits-of-
cinnamon Retrieved on 9/20/18

[86] Cloves: https://www.organicfacts.net/health-benefits/herbs-and-
spices/health-benefits-of-cloves.html Retrieved on 9/20/18

[87] Glucosinolates: https://en.wikipedia.org/wiki/Glucosinolate Retrieved on 8/20/18 * https://en.wikipedia.org/wiki/Isothiocyanate Retrieved on 8/20/18 * https://en.wikipedia.org/wiki/Indoles Retrieved on 8/20/18

[88] Garlic: https://www.webmd.com/vitamins/ai/ingredientmono-300/garlic Retrieved on 9/18/18

[89] Carvacrol: https://en.wikipedia.org/wiki/Carvacrol Retrieved on 8/20/18

[90] Oregano: https://www.naturalfoodseries.com/9-health-benefits-oregano/ Retrieved on 9/18/18

[91] Carnosol: https://en.wikipedia.org/wiki/Carnosol Retrieved on 8/20/18

[92] Betulinic acid: https://en.wikipedia.org/wiki/Betulinic_acid Retrieved on 8/20/18

[93] Rosemary: http://www.whfoods.com/genpage.php?tname=foodspice&dbid=75 Retrieved on 9/18/18

[94] Perillyl alcohol: https://en.wikipedia.org/wiki/Perillyl_Alcohol Retrieved on 8/20/18

[95] Sage: https://www.webmd.com/vitamins/ai/ingredientmono-504/sage Retrieved on 9/18/18

[96] Curcumin: https://en.wikipedia.org/wiki/Curcumin Retrieved on 8/20/18

[97] Piperine: https://en.wikipedia.org/wiki/Piperine Retrieved on 9/12/18

[98] Black pepper: https://draxe.com/peppercorns/ Retrieved on 9/12/18

[99] Capsaicin: https://en.wikipedia.org/wiki/Capsaicin Retrieved on 8/20/18

[100] Beets: https://nutritiondata.self.com/facts/vegetables-and-vegetable-products/2351/2 Retrieved on 9/12/18

[101] Betalains: https://en.wikipedia.org/wiki/Betalain Retrieved on 8/20/18

[102] Dark chocolate: https://nutritiondata.self.com/facts/sweets/5390/2 Retrieved on 9/12/18

[103] Spirulina: https://nutritiondata.self.com/facts/vegetables-and-vegetable-products/2765/2 Retrieved on 9/12/18

[104] Low Sodium V-8: https://nutritiondata.self.com/facts/vegetables-and-vegetable-products/10452/2 Retrieved on 9/12/18

[105] Complete Protein (the nine essential amino acids): Rohini Nag, https://www.healthkart.com/connect/the-all-essential-amino-acids-foods-list-you-must-know-about/ Retrieved on 8/20/18

[106] Flavonoids: https://en.wikipedia.org/wiki/Flavonoid Retrieved on 8/20/18 * https://en.wikipedia.org/wiki/Isoflavonoid Retrieved on 8/20/18

[107] Ginger root: https://www.healthline.com/nutrition/11-proven-benefits-of-ginger Retrieved on 9/18/18

[108] Iodine: https://draxe.com/iodine-rich-foods/ Retrieved on 7/26-18 * https://www.myfooddata.com/articles/natural-foods-high-in-iodine.php Retrieved on 7/26-18

[109] Omega-6 fatty acids: https://draxe.com/omega-6/ Retrieved on 8/20/18

[110] Phytoestrogens: https://en.wikipedia.org/wiki/Phytoestrogen Retrieved on 8/20/18

[111] Sodium: https://draxe.com/low-potassium/ Retrieved on 8/23/18

[112] Pomegranate: https://www.bbcgoodfood.com/howto/guide/health-benefits-pomegranate Retrieved on 9/18/18

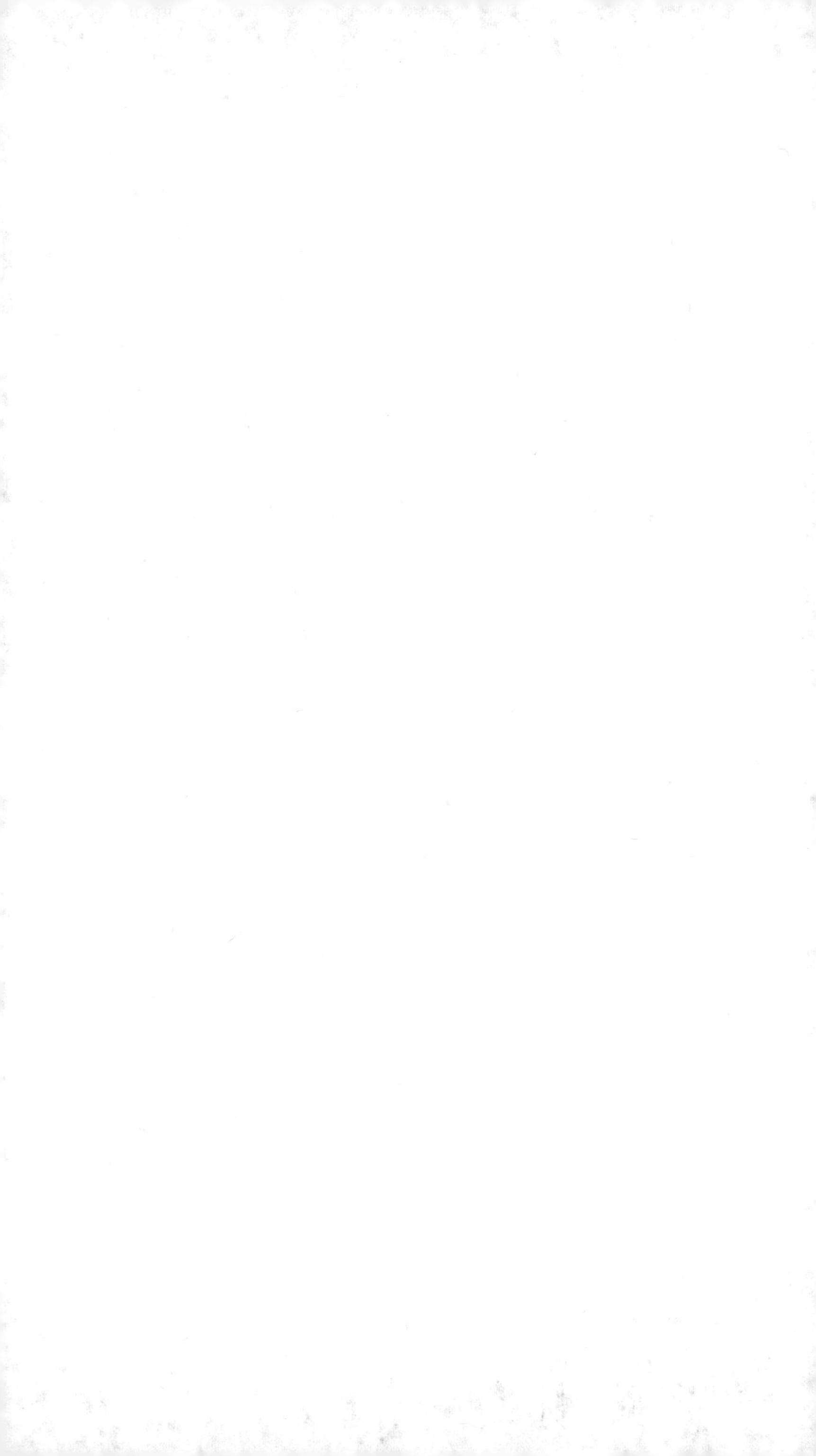